POWER
BRAIN
KIDS

POWER BRAIN KIDS

12 Easy Lessons to Ignite Your Child's Potential

ILCHI LEE

Healing Society

Healing Society

6560 Highway 179, Ste. 114
Sedona, AZ 86351
www.healingsociety.com
1-877-504-1106

First paperback edition: June 2007
Library of Congress Control Number: 2006939644

ISBN: 978-1-935127-35-2

If you are unable to order this book from your local bookseller, you may order through www.amazon.com or www.healingsociety.com.

To *Bella,* whose parents, *Sung* and *Angela,*
are my beloved students and partners

Your children are not your children.
They are the sons and daughters of Life's longing for itself.
They come through you but not from you.
And though they are with you, yet they belong not to you.
You may give them your love but not your thoughts,
For they have their own thoughts.
You may house their bodies but not their souls,
For their souls dwell in the house of tomorrow,
Which you cannot visit, not even in your dreams.
You may strive to be like them, but seek not to make them like you,
For life goes not backward nor tarries with yesterday.
You are the bows from which your children as living arrows are sent forth.
The archer sees the mark upon the path of the infinite,
and He bends you with His might that His arrows might go swift and far.
Let your bending in the archer's hand be for gladness;
For even as He loves the arrow that flies,
so He loves also the bow that is stable.

Kahlil Gibran, from **The Prophet**

Contents

7

Preface

When I was a child, I had a hard time focusing on whatever I was supposed to be doing. Because I was so curious about the world, my mind would wander away from my schoolwork and out into the wider world. After school, I would run to the hills near my home, sit down under my favorite tree, and play with my imaginary friends for the rest of the afternoon.

As a result, my grades suffered, and I frustrated my teachers immensely. Some even told me that I was a "bad boy." However, I was not discouraged by their words. Even though I was very young at that time, I instinctively knew that there was something great in my mind and that I was not a "bad boy" at all. My father agreed and assured me that I would become something great someday. This self-confidence is the greatest gift that I have ever received. As parents and educators, we have the opportunity to give this same gift to the present generation of children.

If we are to instill genuine confidence in our children, we must first have confidence in them. I truly believe that every child's brain has extraordinary potential to create health, happiness, and peace in the world. Don't underestimate and limit your children's potential with typical preconceptions and judgments. Greatness is not limited to those who perform well on standardized tests or to those who know how to sit still at age eight.

Learn to see your children's struggles and difficulties as part of the natural process of becoming the uniquely talented people they are meant to become. Always believe in your children and help them to trust and respect themselves. Help them to discover the great gifts hidden beneath the surface. Let them know that they have great power to choose the conditions and circumstances of their lives. Remind them often that they can do anything that they choose to do.

We adults are responsible for providing the foundation upon which our children may build successful and fulfilling lives. I believe that the optimal development and function of the human brain should be at the core of this foundation. This is why I have dedicated my life to the development of the brain in the hope of uncovering its full potential. During this quest, I have examined everything I could find that has implication for the health of the brain, from the most ancient mind-body practice to the most modern scientific research.

The Brain Education (BE) system reflected in this book is the result of this multidecade search. However, the goal of BE is not to create ideal students and child prodigies. Rather, the intention is to help children gain mastery over their brains as they grow up, giving them an opportunity to fully use their minds toward the creation of their own happiness. As educators and parents, we must ensure that every child views the brain as a boundless resource, a best friend from whom they will never part.

I would like to extend my special thanks to the many BE instructors around the world whose experiences and inspirations have lent so much to the making of this book. Their passionate efforts to bring Brain Education to schools and communities are making the world a better place, one child at a time.

Ilchi Lee
Founder of Brain Education

The Power Brain Concept

Introduction

Wouldn't it be great if we could guarantee our children's happiness? Virtually all parents and educators want to raise children who become highly productive, culturally aware, and emotionally secure adults. Yet so many children head into adolescence and young adulthood filled with angst and doubt about the meaning and direction of their lives.

Realistically, there is no way we can guarantee anyone's happiness, including that of our own children. However, we can provide tools to help them achieve greater happiness on their own. This book, which is based on the Brain Education (BE) training system, places the source of happiness in the brain, not in external things, such as academic or financial success. It is based on the notion that happy, confident people are more likely to be more successful in all areas of life.

Brain-based models of education are becoming increasingly popular, perhaps because today's children will be required to use their brains as no other generation before them. As the population has soared, the human world has in many ways shrunk, bringing people closer together through the technologies of communication and transportation. John Donne said long ago that "no man is an island," but this may be truer today than ever before. In the twenty-first century, one could also contend that "no culture is an island," as peoples merge and interact in ways unique in human history. This trend has brought great blessings and many challenges to the human condition.

Our children do not live in a world where belief systems and bodies of knowledge are passed from generation to generation without external influences. Rather, today's child must face a veritable smorgasbord of information from which to choose. Our children must be able to adapt and process all this varied information easily and peacefully, so that they can make the best choices for themselves and the world as a whole.

For this reason, we must help our children develop brains prepared for this expanded role. Through proper education, the world becomes a treasure trove of possibility for our children, rather than a dreaded Pandora's box of contradictory ideas and misinformation. In the past, educational systems have focused on the storage of facts appropriate to the culture in which they exist.

That approach is no longer adequate in today's complex world. Children must develop skills to make their minds flexible and highly adaptive.

The primary goal of Brain Education is to create "power brains" that are creative, peaceful, and productive. Its intention is not only to make better students but also to create happier, healthier people. While education traditionally emphasizes analytical and verbal skills (consider, for example, the content of the SAT), Brain Education develops interpersonal and intrapersonal skills, as well.

Brain research has clearly established that emotional and physical health directly influence children's ability to learn and consequently affect their performance in school *(see Vail)*. Essentially, the best students are the happiest students. For that reason, Brain Education seeks to enhance learning ability by first creating happier and healthier children. Through consistent BE practice, children gain a sense of empowerment toward the creation of a fulfilling and healthy lifestyle.

Of course, Brain Education is not the only educational system to emphasize the role of the brain in the learning process. Educators are increasingly turning to the discoveries of neuroscience to help them better understand how students learn, and many brain-based educational methods are in use today *(see Nunley)*. In some ways, however, the study of the human brain is still in its infancy, and many aspects of brain function remain a mystery. You could say that we are just now entering "the era of the brain," as neuroscientific knowledge increases almost daily, and the link between this information and educational pedagogy grows stronger and stronger.

The number of academic articles on this topic is staggering, offering research on almost every possible topic, from learning disabilities to gender differences to brain development. The underlying message of all this research is very simple: to understand the child's brain is to understand the child.

I developed the Brain Education method in South Korea in the 1980s as an updating of traditional Korean mind-body health training systems. The principles and practices of the method were then combined with knowledge about the brain gained from neuroscience, psychology, and other fields. Its essential goal, however, remains very straightforward and practical—the physical, emotional, social, and academic betterment of human beings.

Brain Education is currently thriving in hundreds of schools in Korea, and it has recently been successfully introduced in several K–8 schools in the United States. BE curriculum has been especially successful in teaching the

English language to Korean schoolchildren in after-school programs, allowing kids to quickly and easily absorb a language very different from their own. Also, the Korean Institute of Brain Science has hosted two International Brain HSP Olympiads, in which BE-trained children and adults have demonstrated a wide range of advanced mental skills, including information processing, memory, and even extrasensory ability.

Brain Education is especially appropriate for today's children because it offers tools to cope with issues that are unique to the young generation. Children today are sometimes referred to as "Generation M" because media dominate their lives in so many ways. Media technology, such as cable television and the Internet, provides a constant and unlimited flow of information. Youngsters must choose which ideas to accept and which to reject. Their choices in this regard will affect their patterns of thinking about themselves and the world around them. The job of the educator and the parent is to help guide children in making these important decisions, which is a difficult task in a media culture more interested in selling jeans and cola than in creating well-rounded, confident individuals. Brain Education, in its essence, offers simple tools that provide children with the power to choose and use information more effectively.

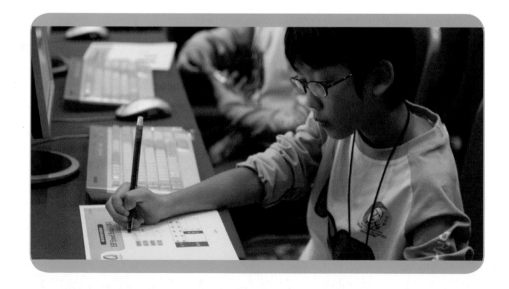

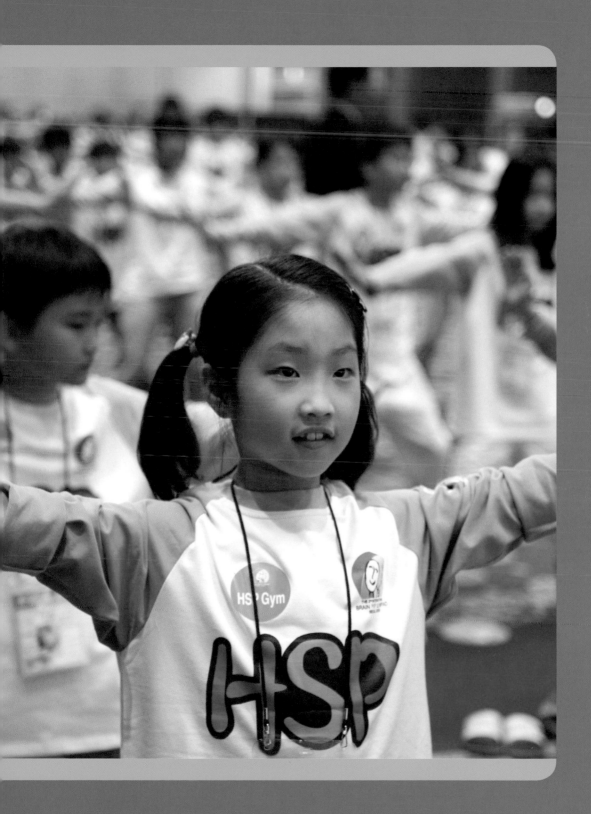

The Five Steps of Brain Education

The process of Brain Education is divided into five steps. As you progress through the twelve lessons, you and your child will move naturally through these five steps. However, perfecting any one of the steps is a lifelong journey, and the skills gained in earlier steps will continue to be utilized in later steps. You will notice that most of the lessons in this book focus on the first and second steps, which are most appropriate for children and beginning practitioners.

Step 1

Brain Sensitizing: Participants become more aware of the brain and its functions. This step may include some basic understanding of brain structure, but more importantly, it creates awareness of the brain as the organ of all perception, especially sensory perception. Furthermore, practitioners can reawaken sensory perception that may have become dulled through habit or environmental overstimulation. The sensitizing process begins with relaxation of body and mind through stretching and breathing exercises. This step primarily corresponds to Lessons 1–3.

Step 2

Brain Versatilizing: During this step, children gain increased flexibility of the brain. Participants learn to shift point of view quickly and to facilitate communication between left and right hemispheres of the brain. This step may include physical exercises that develop coordination, mental exercises that require quick thinking and prolonged concentration, and other activities that develop creativity and imagination. This step primarily corresponds with Lessons 4–7.

Step 3

Brain Refreshing: At this point, children are ready to let go of old, negative information and replace it with positive information about themselves and their surroundings. They learn to control emotions more effectively and to solve problems in a positive manner while overcoming bad habits and debilitating emotions. This process begins with simple awareness of emotions and memories and progresses toward the ability to choose and control emotional states. This step primarily corresponds with Lessons 8–9.

Step 4

Brain Integrating: At this stage, new connections are formed between hemispheres and diverse areas of the brain. The goal is to fully access all layers and connect both hemispheres of the brain for optimal learning and brain functioning. These abilities are then applied to creative problem solving. This step primarily corresponds to Lesson 10.

Step 5

Brain Mastering: Children now fully understand what it means to have a creative, peaceful, and productive "power brain." Equipped with a sense that life is meaningful and purposeful, they are able to maintain a calm, centered way of life most of the time. Although total mastery may not be possible in their lifetime, participants can continue to observe and improve their use of the brain to achieve goals and character growth. This step primarily corresponds to Lessons 11–12.

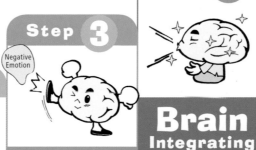
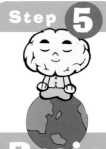
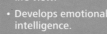

Step 1

Brain Sensitizing

- Awakens the five senses.
- Improves physiological functioning.
- Encourages brain awareness.

Step 2

Brain Versatilizing

- Creates flexibility in brain circuitry.
- Frees brain from rigid habits.
- Opens practitioner to new information.

Step 3

Negative Emotion

Brain Refreshing

- Clears away emotional residue.
- Encourages positive life view.
- Develops emotional intelligence.

Step 4

Brain Integrating

- Unites diverse areas of the brain.
- Enhances communication between hemispheres.
- Releases latent abilities.

Step 5

Brain Mastering

- Empowers authorship of life purpose.
- Enables greater executive control of the brain.
- Expedites decision-making process.

How to Use This Book

In the following pages, you will find a collection of stretching and balancing exercises, followed by the twelve main lessons. The exercises are designed to be used easily by parents with their children, and they can also be readily adapted to classroom use. Most exercises can be followed by a single child, but occasionally there are exercises and games for pairs of children. If working with a single child, an adult can play the second child.

In fact, taking the mind-set of a child is the best approach when working with children using this program. BE instructors are encouraged to "act like seven-year-olds" during their training because that is the best way to ensure an imaginative and accepting mind. So, as you work with your power brain kids, remember to become a kid right along with them. Practice the exercises as they do, making the lessons a fun part of your everyday routine.

Before beginning any Brain Education activities, be sure to do some stretching exercises, like those presented in the Brain-Body Activation section (pages 24–39). When you are lacking time, you may be tempted to skip that, but please don't! These exercises are very critical for circulating oxygenated blood to the brain and for "waking up" the circuitry of the brain. Also, new connections are created in the brain anytime you use the muscles in new ways. So, try to do at least fifteen minutes before beginning any BE activities.

Each of the twelve main Power Brain lessons is designed to be practiced for at least one week before moving on to the next. Each one builds on the skills gained in the previous chapter, so try to complete all lessons in order if possible. However, you may want to try mixing and matching activities to fit the needs of an individual child. You may choose a single five-minute exercise, or you may follow the entire one-hour lesson plan that has been provided. Also, exercises can and should be repeated to increase mastery.

If your schedule is very tight, don't feel pressured to master each lesson completely in a single week. Do try to be regular in practicing the exercises, but be creative in the ways that you integrate this into your family's life. Ideally, you should set aside about an hour to introduce a lesson, but even this can be broken down into manageable segments of time. You will quickly discover that you have more available time than you think for practicing some of these exercises. You can try them while standing in line, riding in the car, or getting ready for bed—any place or time is fine.

Most people find that they are short of "quality time" with their children as they struggle to balance the demands of career and home life. Children, too, have very heavily scheduled lives these days. This may lead to a kind of disconnect between family members. Since many of these exercises are meant to develop both greater self-awareness and sensitivity to the needs of others, use them to connect with your child in a whole new way. And remember, all of these activities are as good for *your* brain as they are for your child's.

As you begin these lessons, it is important to remember that this is a non-traditional educational method. In the past, many educational curricula have focused on the development of specific academic skills, especially verbal and mathematical skills. Brain Education also seeks to develop skills, but many of these skills, such as emotional awareness, creativity, and cooperation, are not easy to measure or quantify in some way. For that reason, it is best to approach these lessons as guided play, rather than as compulsory homework. If your child really does not want to participate, please do not force him or her.

Also, this is not a competitively based educational method. Competitive strategies for student motivation, such as grading and contests, may have their place in certain educational settings, but these are best avoided in beginning Brain Education activities. In fact, many children need a break from highly competitive educational environments, so please allow your child to experience these lessons without that kind of pressure. In the long run, your child will be more prepared for the competitive realities of life if first allowed to gain confidence and self-acceptance.

Last, try to remain positive and patient with your child at all times. Some of the exercises may be difficult at first. Avoid comparing a child's progress to that of other kids, and focus on what he or she is doing well. The important thing is to keep trying! Also, the lessons are designed to be about one hour in length, but the amount of time an individual needs to master particular exercises will vary greatly, so be ready to improvise!

PART 2

Brain-Body Activation

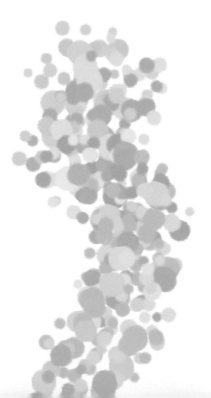

Moving Bodies, Growing Brains

As children become increasingly sedentary in today's technological world, it becomes all the more important for them to make exercise a deliberate and regular part of their daily routine. Research has shown conclusively that movement is essential to a healthy brain since exercise creates the nerve connections needed for optimal brain function *(see Lawrence)*. In addition, it helps to circulate oxygen and nutrients to the brain and stimulates the production of hormones that combat stress and depression.

Just as you guide your children to create healthy habits for nutrition and cleanliness while they are young, guide them also to make physical movement part of their healthy lifestyle. As you may know from your own personal experience, it can be difficult to establish a habit of regular exercise in adulthood. If your child gains this habit now, it will be very firmly established in the actual circuitry of the brain, and he or she will naturally crave physical movement of all types, rather than avoid it as an unappealing chore.

The first section consists of a collection of basic stretching exercises for kids. These yoga-like movements are designed to open up the body's joints, to stretch and strengthen the muscular system, and to promote relaxation. Exercises of this type are wellsuited to brain development because they require the child to use a wide variety of muscles in unique combinations. Any kind of exercise is good, but these are especially effective for creating a balanced and strong bodily structure while at the same time strengthening unity of the mind and body. And kids will become more aware of their own body as they gain flexibility and coordination. If you would like to adapt them to make them fun and appealing to your child, feel free to do so. The important thing is to move!

Standing Postures

Bullfrog Belly

Benefits: Helps intestinal function and releases tension from the abdomen. Allows more circulation to the lower abdomen.

1. Stand with your feet shoulder width apart and your knees bent slightly. Position your hands in the shape of a triangle with your thumbs on your belly button.

2. Push your abdomen out, making your belly round.

3. Pull in your abdomen deeply, keeping your shoulders relaxed. Breathe naturally. Continue to push out and pull in. Repeat 50 times.

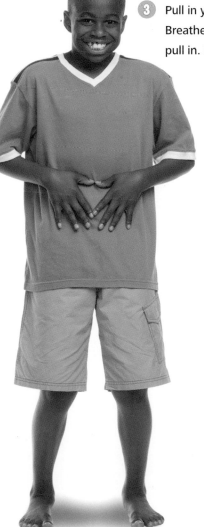

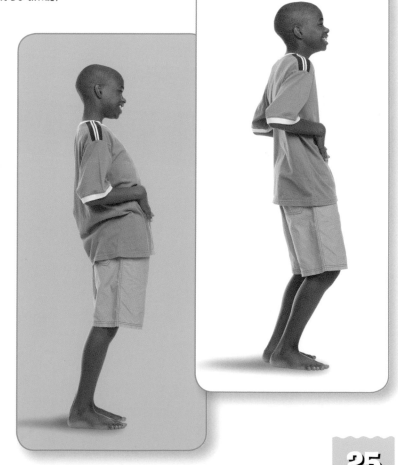

Touching Clouds

Benefits: General, all-over body stretch. Develops balance.

1. Clasp your hands together and push your palms to the ceiling. Inhale as you push. Older children can rise up on tiptoes. Hold for a few counts.

2. Exhale and return to the original position. Repeat 3–5 times.

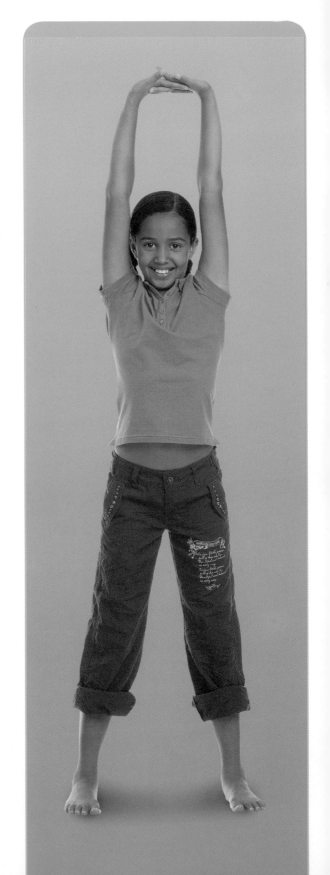

Crescent Moon

Benefits: Stretches the side of the body while increasing circulation to the liver, stomach, and other internal organs.

1. Place your left hand on your waist. Inhale as you reach the right hand over the ear toward the left side. Hold for 3 counts. Exhale and slowly return.

2. Repeat 3 times on each side of the body.

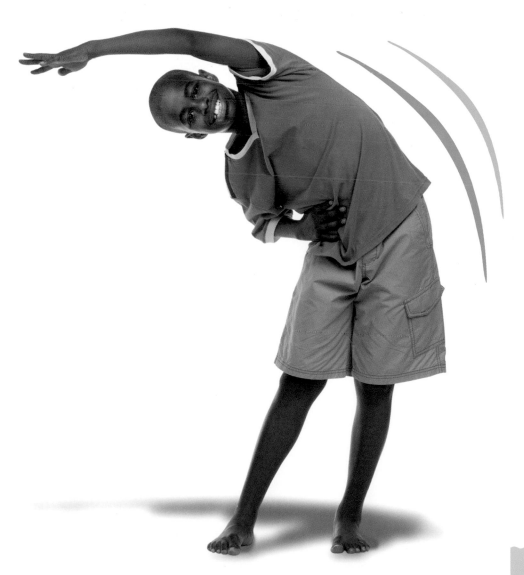

Wringing the Towel

Benefits: Releases tension from the shoulders, while strengthening the shoulder and elbow joints.

1. Stand with your feet apart and hold your arms straight out from your body, parallel to the ground, palms down.

2. As you inhale deeply, twist the hands in opposite directions. Hold for 3 counts. Exhale and return to the original position.

3. Repeat the exercise, switching the direction of the twist. Repeat 3 times in each direction.

Hula Hoop Hips

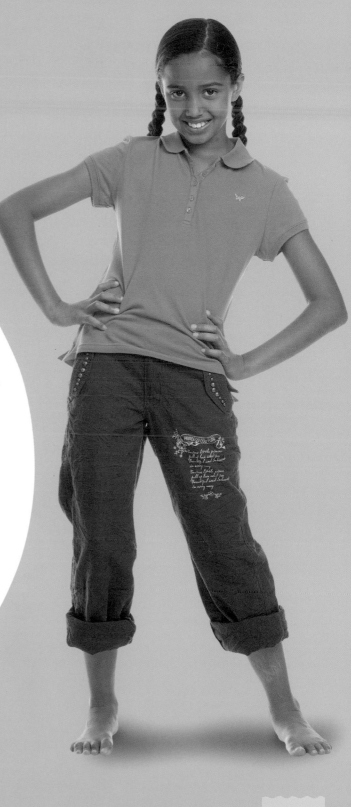

Benefits: Opens the hip joints and releases tension in the lower back.

1 Stand with your feet parallel, shoulder width apart. Place your hands on your hips. Keep your knees straight.

2 Begin to rotate your hips in a large circle, pushing as far as you can in all directions. Repeat 5 times and then reverse and do 5 circles in the opposite direction.

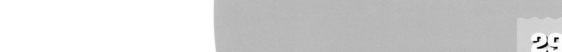

Knee Circles

Benefits: Opens the knee joints and keeps the ligaments pliable. Helps avoid common knee injuries.

1 Stand with your legs straight and feet parallel. Place your hands on your knees.

2 Bend your knees, rotating them in one direction 5 times, and then reverse, making 5 circles in the opposite direction.

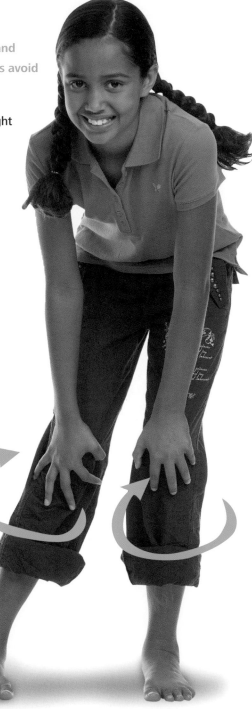

Backward Bow

Benefits: Increases circulation to the spleen and stomach.

1. Place your right foot forward and your right palm on your right thigh.

2. Inhale and reach your left hand back behind your head, your palm facing the ceiling. Let your head drop back as you follow the movement of the hand with your eyes.

3. Exhale and slowly return to the original position.

4. Repeat 3 times and then repeat on the opposite side of the body.

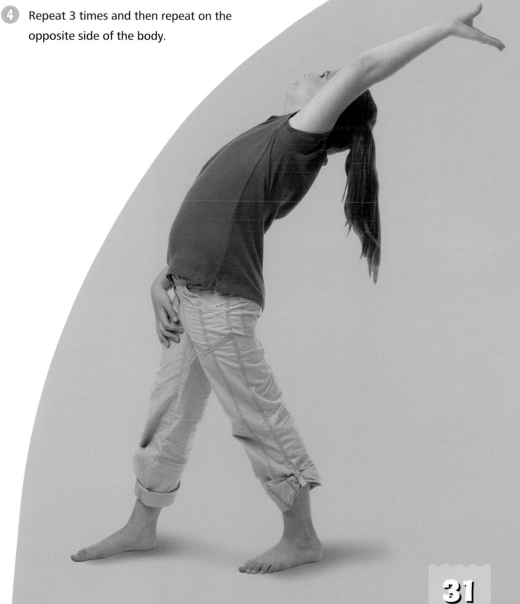

Sitting and Kneeling Postures

Butterfly

Benefits: Opens up the hip joints.

1. Sit on the floor with your back straight. Bring your feet together and your knees out to the side. Hold on to your feet with your hands and bounce your knees several times, relaxing your hip joints.

2. Stop bouncing and straighten your back. Breathe in deeply. Exhale and bring your chest toward your feet. Inhale and straighten up again. Exhale, and relax your shoulders and hips. Repeat 3–5 times.

Little Merman

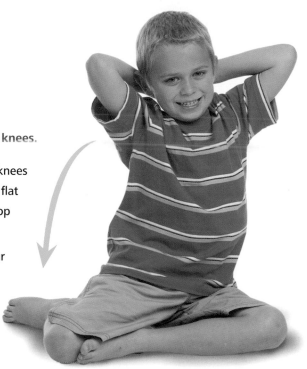

Benefits: Strengthens the hips and knees.

1. While sitting up, bend both knees to the side. Knees should be flat on the ground, not one on top of the other.

2. Clasp your hands behind your head, pushing your elbows out to the side. Now twist your torso opposite to the direction of the bent knees. Bend your torso toward your feet. Hold for three counts. Repeat 3 times and then switch sides.

Stretching Cat

Benefits: Relaxes and realigns the spine and shoulders.

1. Kneel down on the floor. Reach your hands out far in front of you, palms on the ground.

2. Push your hips back and push your face to the ground. Inhale as you pull back your hips. Hold for 5 counts.

3. Exhale and return to the original position. Repeat 5 times.

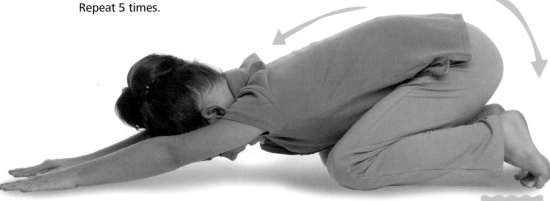

Worried Cat

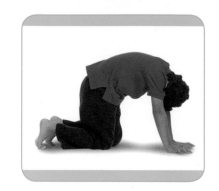

Benefits: Adds flexibility to the spine and purifies the lungs.

1. Kneel with your knees on the ground, palms on the floor. Inhale and round your back up to the sky. Lower your head toward the floor, looking at your abdomen. Pause for 3 counts.

2. Exhale and lower your spine toward the floor. Look up to the ceiling. Repeat 3–5 times.

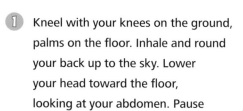

Happy Dog

Benefits: Exercises the waist muscles. Releases tension from the lower back.

1. Kneel with your knees and palms on the floor. Bring your knees together and lift your feet off the ground.

2. Inhale and swing your knees around and look at your feet. Exhale and do the same in the other direction. Repeat 10 times.

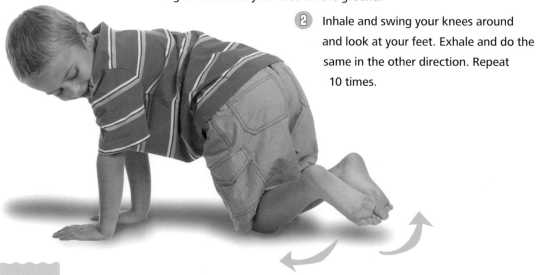

Lying Postures

Barking Sea Lion

Benefits: Adds flexibility to the spine. Stimulates and cleanses the kidneys.

1. Lie face down on the floor. Place your hands beneath your shoulders and inhale as you push up.

2. Look up to the ceiling, keeping the abdomen on the floor. Hold for 5 counts.

3. Exhale and return to the original position. Repeat 3 times.

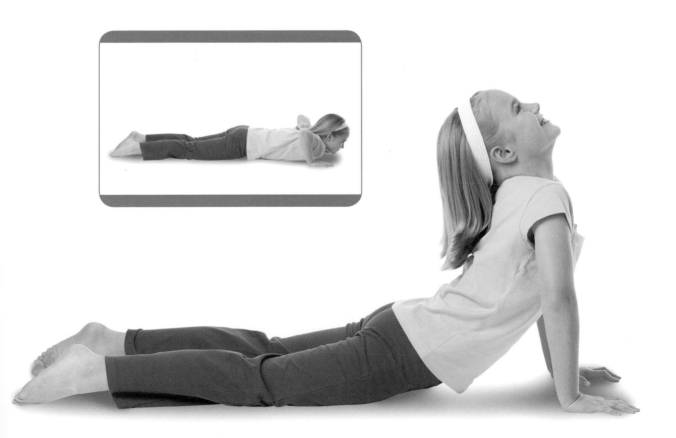

Flip-up Toe Touch

Benefits: Stretches the spine and massages the internal organs. Generally improves circulation.

1. While lying on your back, push your legs and feet up into the air, supporting the weight of your body with your arms and hands. Make your body as straight as possible.

2. Slowly lower your feet to the ground behind your head. Keep your knees straight, bending only at the hips. Hold for ten counts and return.

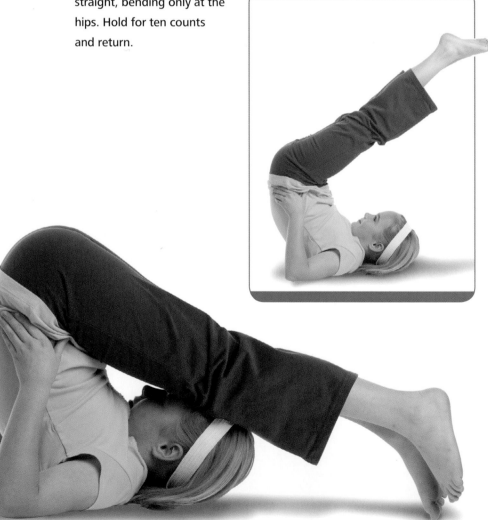

Hip-ups

Benefits: Strengthens the lower back and cleanses the kidneys.

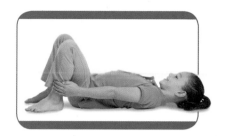

1. Lie on the floor and bend your knees so that your heels are close to your hips, but keep your feet on the floor. Grab your ankles and push your hips up as high as you can while you inhale. Hold for 3 counts.

2. Exhale and return your hips to the ground. Repeat 3–5 times.

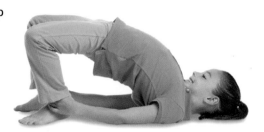

Wriggling Fish

Benefits: Strengthens and tones the muscles in the waist. Quickly improves circulation throughout the body.

1. While lying on the ground, clasp your hands and reach your arms above your head. Put your feet together and point your toes down.

2. Bend your body from side to side. Repeat 10–20 times, changing direction quickly and smoothly.

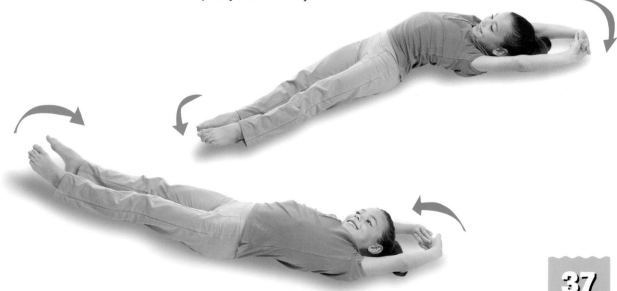

Partner Exercises

London Bridge

Benefits: Opens the shoulders and lower back. Releases stagnant energy from the chest and lungs.

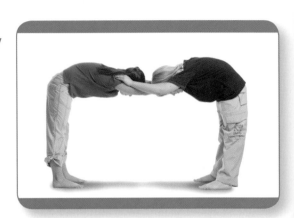

1. Place your hands on the shoulders of your partner. Move your feet back as you bend your body forward. Both partners should bend forward, making a 90-degree angle at the waist.

2. Now, bounce your arms and torso down, counting up to 10. Keep your legs straight.

3. Twist your arms and waist to one side, and bounce 10 times again. Repeat on the other side.

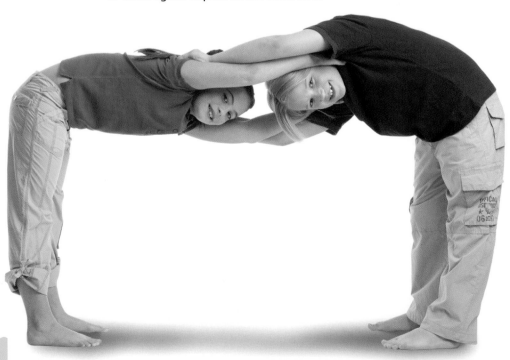

Wheelbarrow

Benefits: Strengthens the arms, shoulders, and back. Builds physical power.

1 Holds on to your partner's ankles. The "wheelbarrow" straightens his or her body and walks forward on the hands.

2 Switch roles and repeat.

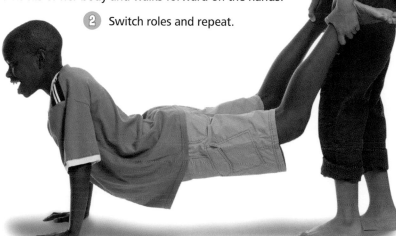

Tandem Bicycle

Benefits: Keeps the hip and knee joints limber. Develops the ability to cooperate with other people.

1 Lie on the floor with the bottoms of your feet against the feet of your partner. Your knees should be bent 90 degrees, and the weight of your legs should rest comfortably against your partner's feet.

2 Begin to make large, slow circles with your feet. Reverse and try to "pedal" backward. Make sure that the circle stays round. Count 20 times in each direction.

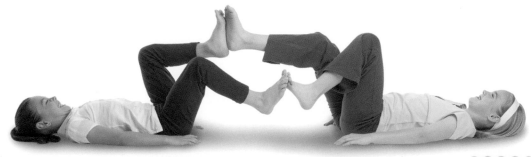

PART 3

Twelve Power Brain Lessons

The Journey Begins

Welcome to your Power Brain journey. As you and your child work through these lessons together, you will have many opportunities to smile and laugh together. Some activities will be very familiar to you, while others may seem unusual. Some exercises will be easy to accomplish, and others may elicit great frustration. Regardless of whatever tasks are at hand, please face them with an open and positive mind. And, of course, always have fun.

Also, don't let your child's Power Brain experience end simply because you've completed the day's lesson and have closed the book. Rather, let these lessons be integrated into your child's daily routine. Stuck at a stoplight? Why not practice the Itsy Bitsy Brainy exercise (page 67) with your child? Has your family's favorite TV show gone to commercials? How about doing the Pill Bug (page 63) or some other Brain-Body Activation exercises (pages 24–39) together? The way you choose to integrate these lessons into your child's life is limited only by your imagination and creativity.

Finally, always remember to "surprise your brain." Easy, familiar tasks do not offer the best stimulation for your brain or that of your child. Tasks that are awkward at first are in fact the ones that create more new connections in your brain. So always be persistent in the mastery of these activities, and deliberately seek out new challenges for your brain. What would you really like to do with your brain that you have never done before? Find out those things and be confident that your brain can master them, even if it does not come easily to you. Develop the habits of a brain-centered lifestyle for your family, always looking for new experiences and new challenges for your brain and that of your child. This is the simple and fun way to build brains to last a lifetime.

Body and Brain Check-up

This check-up will help you determine your child's current condition and will help you assess progress. Perform the following exercises and record the total point value. To prepare the child's body for the test, complete at least fifteen minutes of Brain-Body Activation exercises (pages 24–39) before beginning. After the twelve-week program, retest your child to determine progress.

1 **Hamstring Stretch**

Stand up straight with your feet together. Keep your knees completely straight and bend forward at the waist. Try to touch the floor with your hands. Which describes your ability?

- **1** point: Fingers do not touch the floor.
- **2** points: Fingertips touch the floor.
- **3** points: Palms touch the floor.

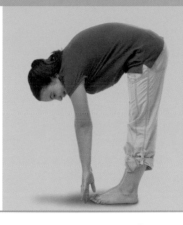

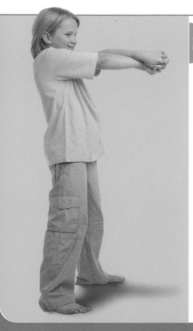

2 **Wrist Twist**

Extend your left arm straight out in front of your chest and twist your wrist so that it faces outward toward the left. Place your right palm on the left palm and clasp your hands together. Keeping your palms tightly clasped, bring your hands down toward your abdomen, bending your elbows. Then lift your clasped hands up through your arms and extend them out as straight as you can. Which best describes you?

- **1** point: I cannot straighten my arms.
- **2** points: I can straighten my arms, but it is painful.
- **3** points: I can easily straighten my arms.

3 Balance Check

Extend your arms out to the side, and lift one foot up so that it is even with your knee. Count slowly to 10. Repeat on the other side. Now, try again, but with your eyes closed. How did you do?

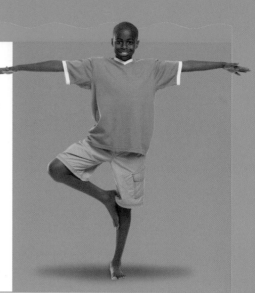

1 point: I have a hard time balancing for the full 10 counts.

2 points: I balance easily with eyes open, but not with eyes closed.

3 points: I can balance well, either way.

4 Mind-Body Check

Curl your right hand into a fist and lightly tap your chest. At the same time, repeatedly sweep your chest with your left palm. Continue for a few seconds, then switch, sweeping with your right palm and tapping with your left fist. Switch one more time. Was this easy for you?

1 point: It is hard to do the exercise at all.

2 points: I can easily do the two motions, but it is hard to switch.

3 points: I can easily do the two motions at the same time, and it is easy to switch.

5 Strength Check

Take the posture for a full BE Push-up (page 49), with arms and body completely straight. Hold the posture for as long as you can, without moving your body. How long did you keep the posture?

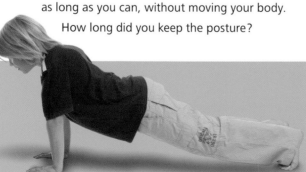

1 point: I cannot hold the posture for a full minute.

2 points: I can hold the posture for 1–2 minutes.

3 points: I can hold the posture for more than 2 minutes.

Extra credit – Add 1 point for each additional minute.

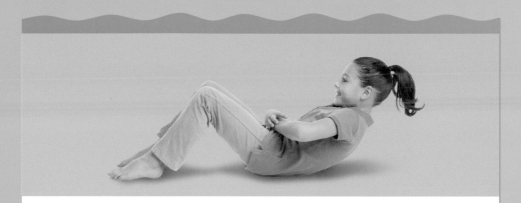

6 Endurance Check

Following the correct Sit-up posture (page 50), complete as many sit-ups as possible. Make sure your feet stay on the floor. How many did you do?

1 point: Less than 10

2 points: 10–20

3 points: 20–30

Extra credit – Add 1 point for each additional set of 10 sit-ups.

7 Power Check

Assume the Sleeping Tiger posture pictured below (page 51). Hold the posture for as long as possible without moving your body. How long can you hold this posture?

1 point: Less than 5 minutes.

2 points: 5–10 minutes.

3 points: More than 10 minutes.

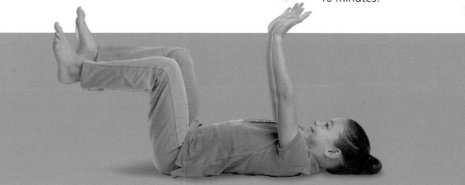

Total points:

Week 12 retest:

Lesson 1

Physical Strength

As you look at the content of this lesson, you may wonder, "Where are the brain exercises?" You may have expected brain teasers and games to challenge your child's mind. Yet all of the activities in this lesson are simple physical exercises, not unlike what you would find in a traditional gym class. In actuality, it stimulates the brain because all movement requires intricate coordination between the body and the brain, which helps to create new brain connections. Also, the increased blood flow to the brain that results helps to nourish and sustain the overall health of the brain.

The body is essentially the brain's connection to the outside world. A person's brain can have little effect on the surrounding environment if the rest of the body lacks strength and stamina. And the condition of the body drastically affects the functioning of the brain. A sluggish, tired body usually equates with a sluggish, tired brain. A strong, vibrant body generally houses a strong, vibrant brain.

For that reason, the goal of strengthening the body should go hand in hand with the goal of strengthening the brain. Sitting behind a desk studying a book is a great way to gather piles of facts and figures, but it will do little to create new and stronger connections in the brain. Rather, this happens through overcoming physical challenges and developing new skills.

Make physical exercise a normal and natural part of your child's daily routine. Children who spend the day watching TV or sitting in front of a computer monitor are being deprived of the chance to develop brain connections that will be much harder to develop later in life. Also, the sense of confidence and accomplishment that comes with physical strengthening will be invaluable to them in many areas of life.

Strength Builders:

The following exercises should be practiced daily during the twelve-week lesson plan. Record the child's progress in a journal or notebook, and try to add more time or repetitions every day, creating goals that are realistic for your child's physical condition.

Tummy Tapping

This may seem to be a slightly unusual exercise, but it is highly effective for stimulating blood circulation and helping to carry the brain's chemical messengers throughout the body. It can also improve intestine function. Begin with 100 repetitions and work up to 500.

1 Stand up straight with your feet shoulder width apart. Bend your knees slightly and place your hands on your abdomen, right below your belly button.

2 Cup your hands slightly and begin to pat firmly on the lower abdomen.

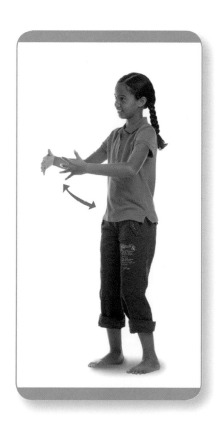

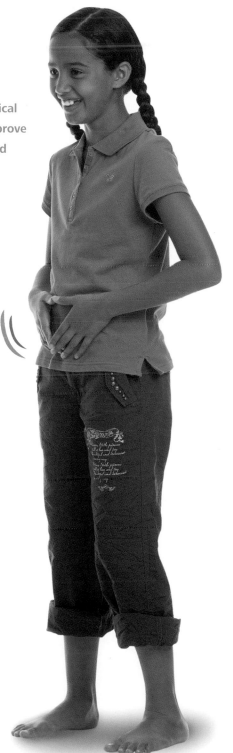

Reach and Squat

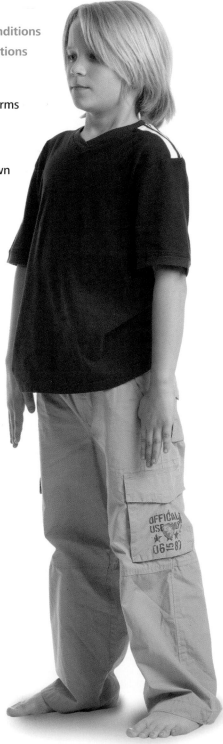

This exercise builds strength in the legs and conditions the cardiovascular system. Begin with 10 repetitions and work up to 100.

1. Begin by standing straight up with your arms straight at your sides, your palms facing the rear.

2. Bend your knees and lower your hips down as low as possible without lifting your heels off the ground. Reach your hands forward as you lower your hips. Keep your back as straight as possible.

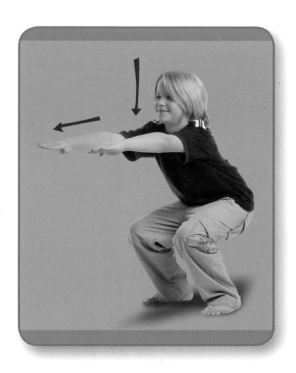

BE Push-ups

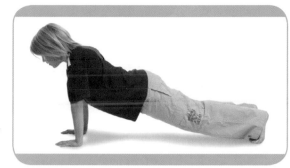

Push-ups are an old-fashioned exercise, but their benefit remains as real as ever. In addition, they require no special equipment and can be done just about anywhere. If they practice them regularly, children can improve quickly, gaining confidence in their physical body, even if they are not considered "athletic." If a child cannot perform a full-position push-up at first, try the alternate position and work up to a full push-up. When a child can perform 100 knee push-ups without stopping, try the full-position posture.

1 Place the palms on the floor, directly under the shoulders. Keep the body perfectly straight as you push your body off the floor. Look forward and keep your feet together.

2 Bend your elbows at a 90-degree angle as you lower your body to the floor. Keep your back and legs straight.

3 Push back up to the starting position and repeat.

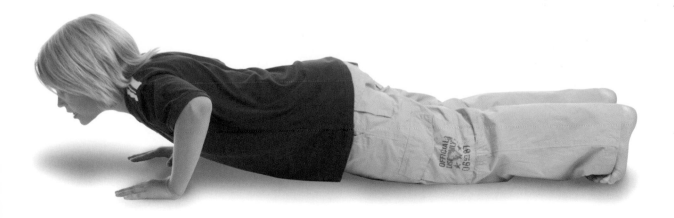

Alternative: Keep the back straight, but place the knees on the floor.

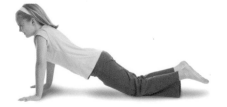

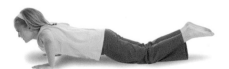

BE Sit-ups

This is another classic exercise that is great for strengthening the body. It helps to build the abdominal "core" of the body. Also, kids can quickly increase the number of sit-ups they can do, thus generating confidence and a sense of accomplishment. Follow the proper position to build genuine strength without risking injury. You may wish to begin by holding the child's feet down, but eventually the child should complete the exercise without this assistance.

1. Lie on the floor and bend your knees at a 90-degree angle. Keep your hands on your lower abdomen.
2. Lift your chest to an upright position, keeping your feet on the floor and your palms on your abdomen.
3. Return to the original position and repeat.

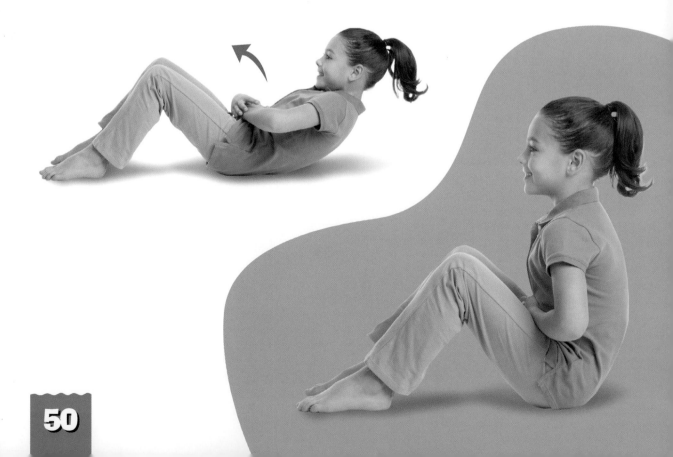

Sleeping Tiger Power Builder

This posture also helps to build core strength, which lies in the lower abdomen area. Most physical exercises will help to build core strength to a certain extent, but this exercise is particularly effective and easy to follow. If core strength is weak, this posture may be difficult at first, but keep trying! Practice this exercise every day, working up to a 15 minutes.

1. Lie comfortably on the floor.

2. Lift your arms straight into the air with your palms facing the ceiling. Flex your wrists back, but don't lock your elbows.

3. Lift your legs off the ground, creating 90-degree angles at the hips and knee joints. Keep your legs parallel and parted shoulder width.

4. Flex you ankles so that your toes are pulled slightly back toward your head. Hold the posture as long as possible.

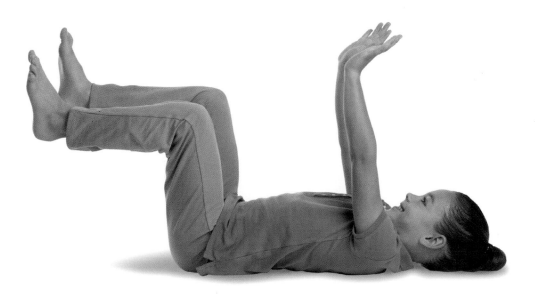

Basic Brain Awareness

The human brain is an amazing organ. It is in charge of all our physical functions, and it is the source of all our emotions and thoughts. All human creations—our art, our architecture, our technologies—begin with the brain. Our brains, in fact, are what make us essentially human. The unique abilities of the human brain are what most clearly separate us from apes, and it is our brain, not brawn, that has established our predominate role on the planet. Our physical bodies, while amazing in their own right, are relatively weak. We have no fangs or talons, and even the most developed human musculature pales compared to that of a grizzly or an ox. Nevertheless, we thrive as no other animal has thrived on this planet. Why? Because the brain has allowed us to control and adapt the environment to suit our needs, delivering us from many of the harsher realities of nature.

Yet, like adults, kids are often unaware of the importance of the brain. Try asking a kid, "What is the most important organ?" The child might respond, "The heart." Or she might say, "The lungs." But the truest answer is definitely "The brain." After all, none of those organs can function without the guidance of the brain. Yet, when people speak of health in general, the brain is often neglected. It is almost as if the brain is so busy looking around at other things, analyzing and problem solving, that it forgets to look at itself!

That is why a child's Power Brain journey should begin with a basic understanding of the brain and its functions. There is no need for detailed, in-depth knowledge. Many aspects of the brain, in fact, remain a mystery to even the most accomplished neuroscientist. Rather, children need just enough understanding to help them visualize and appreciate how the brain works.

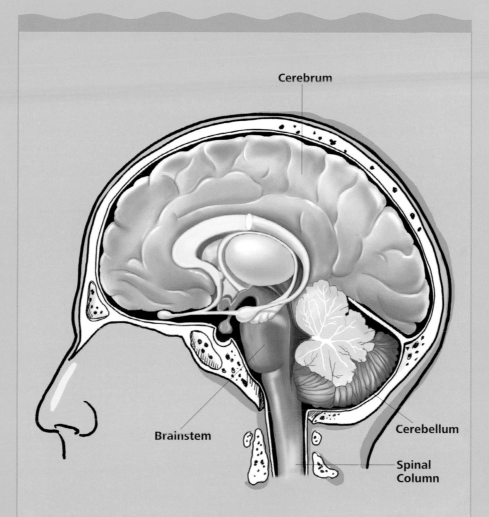

Cerebrum

Brainstem

Cerebellum

Spinal
Column

For the purposes of this book, we focus on only four parts of the brain—the cerebrum, brainstem, cerebellum, and spinal column. There are many other lobes and parts of the brain, but this information may be overwhelming to present all at once. Basic knowledge of the **spinal column** helps children become aware of how all parts of their body are connected to their brain. The **brainstem** is significant because it works independently of the conscious brain, regulating heartbeat, breathing, and other basic bodily functions. The role of the **cerebellum** in coordinating balance and bodily movement helps kids become aware of how their brains help them walk, run, and play. Finally, the **cerebrum** is the thinking part of the brain, the part that processes new ideas, decides how and when to move, and interacts with the rest of the world.

Play-doh Brains

This activity will help children concretely understand the basic structure and function of the brain. In addition, working with modeling compound helps to build dexterity. Follow each step, but don't worry about the results looking perfect. Supply a simple picture of the brain, such as the one provided on page 53, to help children understand the various parts in relation to the others.

1. Roll a small Play-doh "worm" to represent the spinal column. Explain that the spinal column connects our brain to the rest of our bodies.

2. Create a pea-sized Play-dohball in a different color. Connect the ball to the top of the Play-doh spinal column. Explain that it represents the brainstem, which controls involuntary bodily functions, like heart beat, breathing, digestion, etc.

3. Make three Play-doh balls in different colors. Two balls, which represent the two halves of the cerebrum, should be the size of two large gumballs, while the cerebellum is represented by a ball the size of a small gumball. Join the parts together with the other structures to form a complete brain. Explain how the cerebellum (the small gumball) helps us keep our balance and move our bodies, and the two large halves of the cerebrum help us think, create, speak, and learn.

Body and Brain Relaxation

This activity will help reinforce what was learned about the brain and will help children use that information to visualize the brain. It will also help them release tension from the body.

1. Lie down on the floor, arms to the side and legs on the ground. Position your legs shoulder width and bring your arms forty-five degrees from the body, palms facing the ceiling. If this is not possible, sit comfortably, arms relaxed with palms facing upward. Close your eyes, feeling your chest fill with air as you breathe in. Slowly exhale, feeling the air come slowly out of your mouth.

2. Relax each part of the body as you call out its name. Begin with the face, feeling the forehead, eyes, jaw, and mouth releasing tension. Feel your neck relax. Release tension from the shoulders. Allow the chest to expand more and more as you breathe. Relax the abdomen, thighs, calves, and feet.

3. Continue breathing as you imagine oxygen traveling farther up the spinal column with each breath. Imagine each part of the brain lighting up like a light bulb as oxygen reaches it. Call out each part of the brain as it begins to glow.

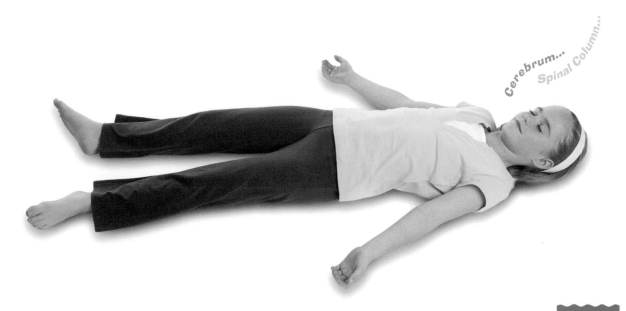

Cerebrum... Spinal Column...

Brain Watching and Drawing

In this exercise, kids can become familiar with their own brain. Also, it develops focus, imagination, and self-awareness. Don't worry about whether or not kids visualize the brain with anatomical perfection. This activity should be done directly after Body and Brain Relaxation so that no tension is held in the body.

1. Sit comfortably. Place your hands on your knees with the palms facing the ceiling. Straighten your back. Relax all the muscles of the body.

2. Visualize the outside of the head first. Ask, "What does your head look like from above?"

3. Then go deeper into the head, imagining the shape of the brain. Ask, "What does your cerebrum look like? What is its shape? What color is it? What is it doing right now?"

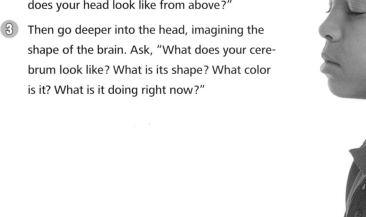

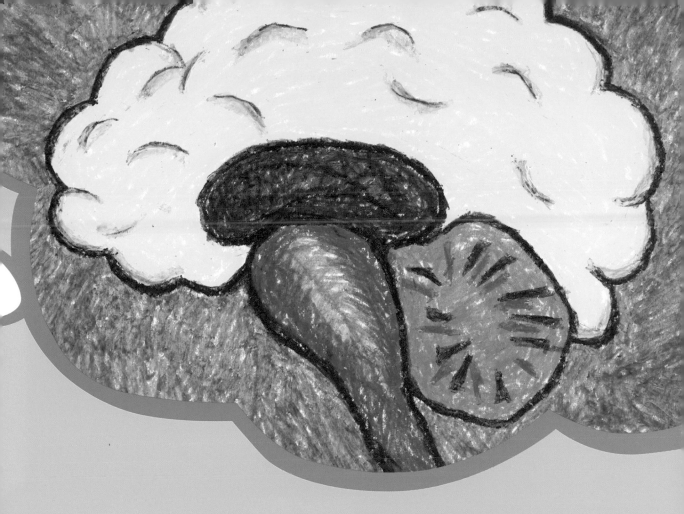

4 Do the same for each part of the brain—cerebellum, brainstem, and spinal column.

5 Slowly open your eyes.

6 Now draw your brain. Show all the different colors and shapes. You can use whatever colors and shapes best represent you. Explain your drawing to your parent or a friend.

What **COLOR** is your brain? What shape is your brain?

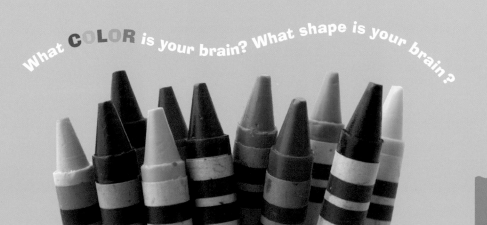

Body-Brain Awareness

Children may not be aware at first that the brain either consciously or unconsciously controls everything that they do and feel. Tickle a child's foot and ask him, "Where do you feel the tickle?" The child will probably say, "On my foot." This is a chance to explain to the child how the brain is the place where the tickle is actually felt. If the foot is removed from the body, it can no longer send the tickle message to the brain. Likewise, all the body's organs and muscles are connected to the brain, following its commands.

While it is true that the brain is "in charge" of the human body, it can also be said that the brain is useless without the body. The brain gives the orders, but it is the body that puts these orders into action. Sometimes, we are not in conscious control of these actions—as in the beating of the heart or breathing while we sleep—but for the most part we have conscious control over our bodies' movements. We can control our bodies because we can control our brains.

It is important, therefore, that children have a good basic understanding of the body and its functions. It is helpful to speak of the various organs of the body as "little brains," organs that are in charge of specialized functions within the body. Through familiarity with various organs and their connection to the brain, children gain the ability to take charge of the body and its overall state of health.

Little Brain Game:

This game requires quick thinking, and it will help kids learn the locations of organs in the body. Begin by explaining the basic function and location of the lungs, heart, stomach, kidneys, and liver. Have kids place their hands on each location.

- The **lungs** bring oxygen to the blood every time you breathe.

- The **heart** pumps oxygenated blood throughout the body.

- The **stomach** uses acids and enzymes to break down food to make energy for your body.

- The **kidneys** filter blood to remove excess liquid and wastes.

- The **liver** removes toxic substances from the blood.

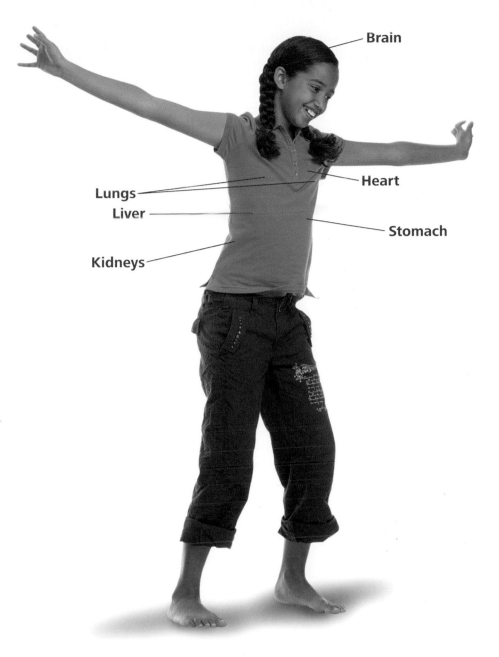

Brain

Heart

Lungs

Liver

Stomach

Kidneys

Instruct children to place their hands on the organ that you call out. Once they are proficient, place your hand in a place other than what you named. For example, call out "liver" and then place your hand on the kidneys. See how fast they can find the correct organ.

Now make it harder by doing it in groups. Tap one organ three times, and then call out another. Place your hand on the wrong spot on the body when you call out the last item. Call out, for example, "Liver, liver, liver, stomach" but place your hand on your heart. See if they can follow your words, not your movements.

"Little Brain" Exercises:

These postures stimulate energy and blood circulation to the various major organs of the body. They are based on the system of energy pathways used by acupuncturists to promote health and to treat diseases. Theoretically, if an energy pathway related to a particular organ is completely open, it will ensure total health in that organ. These exercises help open energy pathways related to the specific organs.

Breathing Tiger (for the liver)

This posture is similar to the Sleeping Tiger in Lesson 1 (page 51). Try to hold the correct angles in the body throughout the exercise.

1. Lie down on the ground and relax your body completely.

2. Lift your legs off the ground, bending the knees and ankles at 90-degree angles. Keep your hands on your lower abdomen. Relax your shoulders and arms.

3. Breathe in deeply to the abdomen, causing the belly to expand. Exhale slowly, deflating your abdomen. Breathe in and out slowly 50 times.

4. Lower your hands and legs. Bring your hands to the liver and feel warmth in the liver area.

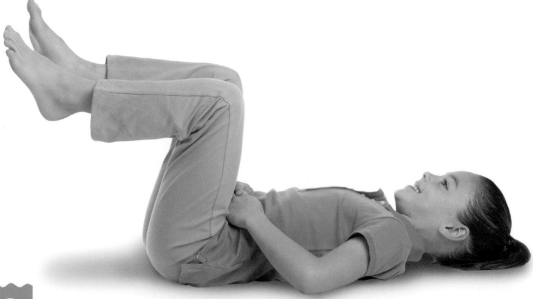

Bow and Arrow (for the heart)

For this one, your child can pretend to be an ancient soldier pulling back a giant, heavy bow. By using imagination and pulling back with full strength, your child will feel greater openness in the chest.

1. Imagine that you are holding a bow in your left hand.

2. Turn your upper body to the left and pull back on the imaginary string with your right hand. Pretend that it is a very heavy bow and difficult to pull back. Tense your muscles, breathe in deeply, and pull back with all your might. If you do this right, your muscles will shake and you might even start to sweat.

3. Exhale and release the bow. Repeat the exercise 5 times.

4. Switch hands and do the same thing on the other side of the body.

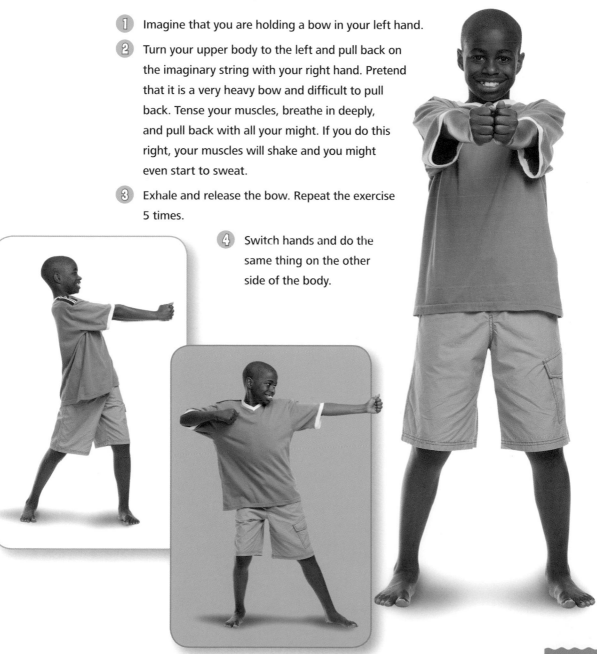

Clapping Machine (for the lungs)

This exercise is a great stress reliever and helps to dissipate negative emotions.

1. Stand with your feet shoulder width apart.

2. Extend your arms straight out in front of you, palms together.

3. Breathe in deeply and push your hands straight back, opening your arms as far as they will go.

4. Exhale quickly and clap your hands. Immediately spring back into the first position, feeling the stretch in the chest and the squeeze in the shoulder blades. Repeat the exercise 10 to 20 times, using large, rapid movements.

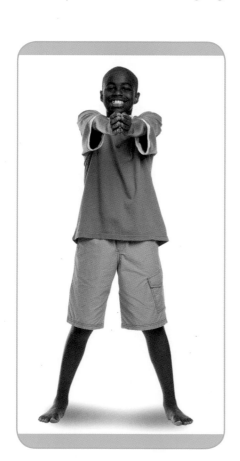

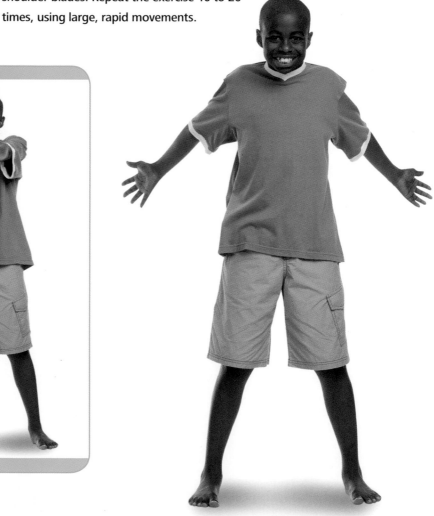

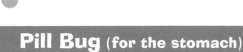

Pill Bug (for the stomach)

This movement is a lot of fun for kids, and it helps to give flexibility to the spine while releasing tension from the stomach. Try it if your child ever has a slight "nervous stomach."

1. Sit on a soft mat, carpeting, or grass and hug your knees. Make your back round.

2. Gently roll backward, from your tailbone to the top of your spine. Roll back again. Repeat 10 to 20 times.

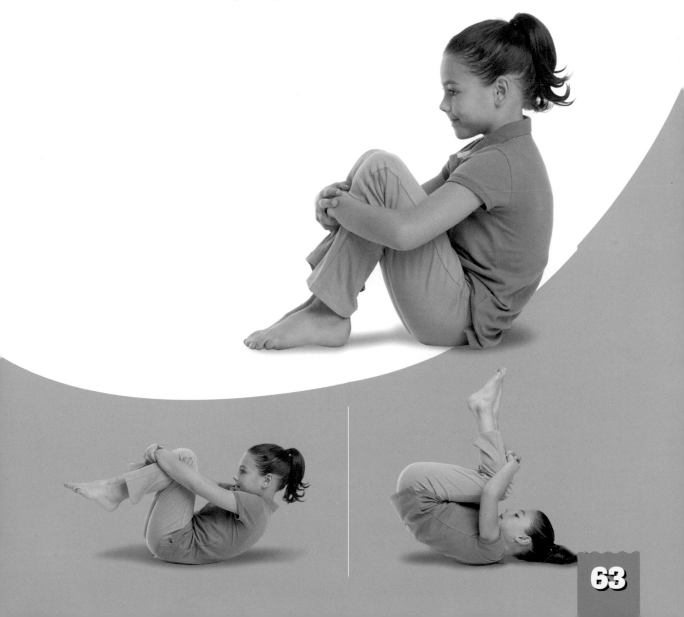

Superman (for the kidneys)

In addition to squeezing and cleansing the kidneys, this exercise helps to strengthen the lower back muscles, which often become weak if your child sits too much.

1. Lie down on your abdomen. Stretch your arms straight out above your head. Breathe in and lift your arms, legs, and chest off the ground. Balance on your abdomen. Hold the posture for 10 counts. Breathe naturally while holding the posture.

2. Exhale and slowly lower your arms and legs to the ground. Repeat 10 times.

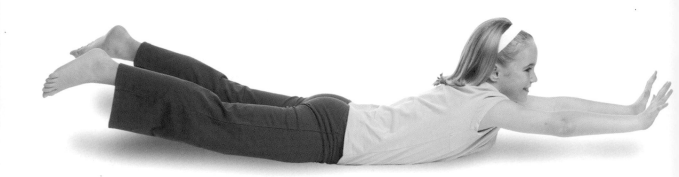

Little Brain Relaxation

This exercise helps children learn to relax deeply while cultivating an appreciative and caring mind toward their body.

1. Lie on the floor or a mat, arms to the sides, palms facing upward, and feet shoulder width apart.

2. Breathe in, focusing on the chest, and slowly breathe out, relaxing the body completely.

3. Bring your hands to each of the five "little brains," one at a time—liver, heart, stomach, kidneys, lungs. In your mind, say, "I love you," to each of the organs. For the kidneys, slide the hands under the lower back.

4. Continue to breathe, and relax the entire body. Feel the warm energy from the hands penetrating into the body.

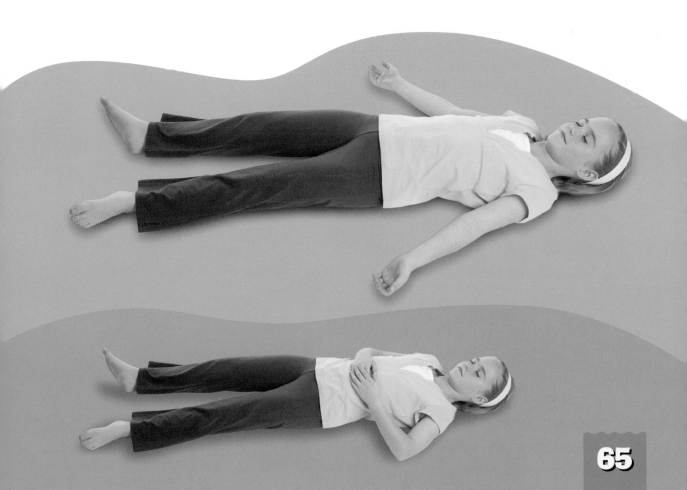

Lesson 4
Brain Balance and Flexibility

Flexibility in the body is an obvious requirement for health. If we cannot move well, we do not feel well. Without flexibility, we lack energy and motivation.

The same can be said of the brain. To function well, it must be flexible, moving from one task to another with ease. Unfortunately, the brain can succumb to limiting habits very easily. Even small children tend to favor that which is "easy," and they avoid things that are "hard." This tendency will often prevent a child from discovering his or her true potential.

For example, a child may decide at a very young age, "I can't sing." To some degree this may be true. Perhaps his or her genetic makeup simply does not include the traits required for genuine musical talent. Maybe he or she is completely tone deaf. But does that mean he or she cannot improve and achieve some level of musical proficiency? Probably not. The child may never be an opera star, or even a suitable member of the local choir, but he or she very likely can gain some musical competence. By deciding not to attempt singing, the child has unconsciously denied the brain the opportunity to develop the complex synaptic connections involved in musicianship.

A truly flexible brain is one that is open and ready to learn and does not avoid the difficult or unusual. The activities in this lesson may be difficult and frustrating at first, but the process of mastering them will build brain connections that facilitate learning and understanding in many areas of life.

As you probably already know, the brain consists of two sides, the left hemisphere and the right hemisphere. One side or the other tends to be dominant, which accounts for left- and right-handedness. In fact, we not only tend to have a dominant hand, but also have a dominant eye and foot. (See *The Dominance Factor* by Carla Hannaford to help determine dominance for yourself or your children.) This is a normal and natural thing, but it can leave the non-dominant side undeveloped and truncate the ability of the left and right sides to communicate. In other words, the brain may be left imbalanced in its development. So try some of these exercises to create more interaction between both sides of your child's brain.

Hand Coordination Exercises

The following exercises help create better communication between left and right sides of the brain by using the left and right hands at the same time. These can be difficult at first, so be patient and practice regularly.

Tap and Sweep:

1. Tap your right fist on the right side of your chest while your left hand sweeps up and down on the left side.

2. Now switch sides, your right hand sweeping and your left fist tapping.

3. See how fast you can switch back and forth.

Itsy Bitsy Brainy:

1. Put your thumbs and index fingers together, as in the game "Itsy Bitsy Spider." Your right index finger should be on your left thumb, and your left index finger on your right thumb.

2. Now, separate the bottom thumb and finger and swing them up over the top thumb and finger, touching them together again. Repeat this action, continuing to "walk" up 5 times.

3. Switch direction and begin to walk the fingers down.

4. Now, begin to walk up again, but this time switch to the middle finger. Walk up and down 5 times, just as before.

5. Continue the same action, switching between fingers. When you reach the pinkie, reverse and work back to the index finger.

67

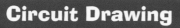

Circuit Drawing

These simple drawing activities provide a couple of very valuable benefits. First, they increase hand-eye coordination, and second, they create a meditative rhythm that helps to soothe and calm the brain waves. Don't forget to switch hands to develop the non-dominant side of the brain.

Infinity Drawing:

This exercise can be used as a calming meditation and to help children focus more clearly.

1. Illustrate to the child what a "lazy eight" infinity symbol looks like.

2. Draw the infinity symbol with a crayon. Preferably, use large paper so the child's whole arm can move, not just the wrist. Keep tracing the symbol for several minutes until the movement is smooth and balanced.

3. Now, switch hands and keep tracing. If you like, switch crayon color. Continue until the movement is smooth and relaxed. Optionally, try drawing the infinity with eyes closed.

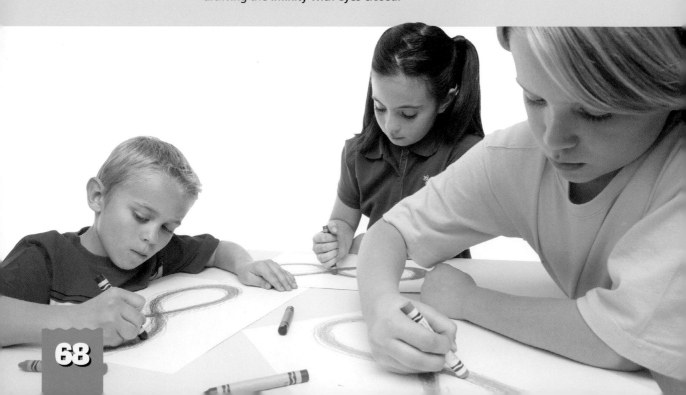

"L" Brain Circuit:

This is a slightly more complicated version of Infinity Drawing, so try it after your child has mastered the preceding exercise.

1. Show children how to draw the figure shown here. Have them draw it on a large piece of paper.

2. Trace the figure up and down, keeping both sides of the figure balanced and even. Switch hands. Keep practicing until the action is smooth and comfortable.

Brain Breathing and Relaxation

Adults sometimes mistakenly think that kids have no experience of stress and tension. This is far from the truth. Kids are under a lot of pressure to compete in school, to maintain a desirable status with their peers, and to live up to parental expectations. To top it off, family situations are often unstable, leaving them with little sense of foundation and centeredness. Doctors report that the incidence of serious anxiety disorders is on the rise, and that now as many as 10 percent of children suffer from these problems.

It is a mistake to wait until adulthood to begin teaching stress management. By this time, negative habits may be very deeply ingrained. As a parent, you might think of yourself as your child's stress-management coach. Very naturally, your child will look to you for ways to cope with the many difficult issues that are part of life.

So, first become a good role model to your children. The ways you choose to handle stress in your own life are likely to be mimicked by your children. If you need to, change the ways you react to stress and find ways to release stress, such as breathing and meditation. If you incorporate these things into your daily life, your children will consider them a normal and natural part of life.

Children often lack the words needed to verbalize the stress they feel, and their physical and emotional symptoms may be very different from an adult's. Physically, children manifest stomachaches and headaches in response to stress, or they may have trouble sleeping. Emotionally, they may be prone to outbursts about seemingly petty things, situations unrelated to the actual cause of stress. Also, you may find that they have become very suddenly shy or introverted.

As with so many human problems, communication offers many solutions for stress. Make it clear to your children that they can talk to you about any problem freely and openly. No matter how small a problem may seem to your adult ears, listen with openness and acceptance. A child may hide a problem if he or she feels it will disappoint you. So demonstrate to your child that your love is unconditional, and that you are honored to help your child in this way. Make it clear that no problem is too small or too embarrassing to be dealt with honestly and sincerely.

Breathing Buddy Exercise

With practice, children can learn to become aware of their breath and develop the habit of deep abdominal breathing, which will be very important for maintaining future health.

1. Lie on your back and relax fully. Place a small stuffed toy on your abdomen, just below the belly button. Part your legs slightly and bring your arms to the side, palms facing upward.

2. Close your eyes and feel the natural rhythm of your breath. Feel your chest gently rising and falling. Let your body relax more and more deeply with each breath.

3. Once your body is fully relaxed, focus on bringing the breath down to the abdomen as your buddy rides up and down. Avoid straining or forcing your abdominal muscles. Continue for at least 5 minutes.

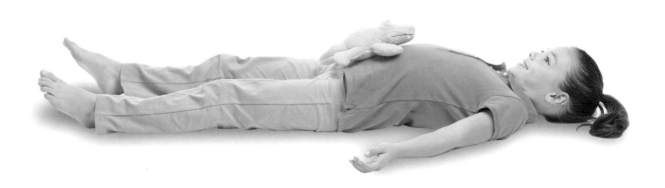

Golden Brain Meditation

This meditation exercise uses deep focus and visualization to help relax and energize the brain. It is also excellent for developing relaxed concentration.

1. Sit comfortably on the floor or in a chair, palms facing upward on your knees or thighs. Close your eyes and focus on the surface of your palms.

2. Keep focusing on your palms, feeling any sensation that is present. You may feel tingling, warmth, or some other sensation. Whatever you feel is fine, as long as you keep focusing on the palms.

3. Now slowly bring your palms off your knees, and hold them about 2–3 inches apart. In your mind's eye, imagine that there is a golden ball of light between your hands. As you breathe in, increase your ball of light as you move your hands more widely, and let it shrink as you exhale.

4. Slowly bring the imaginary ball of light to your head. Visualize the bright energy sinking into the head and into the brain.

5. Return your palms to your knees and focus on your brain. Continue to visualize bright light emanating from within the brain.

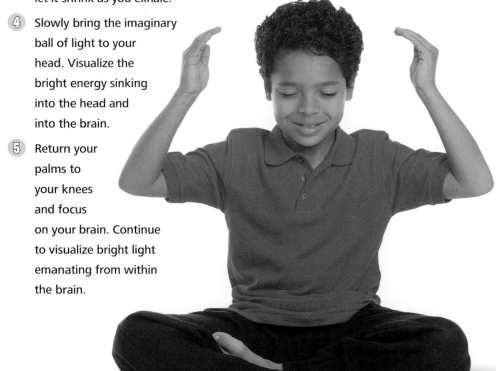

Bright Eyes Exercise

Children can experience great eye fatigue when reading, studying, and working on computers. Make this simple exercise part of your routine in order to avoid eye problems.

1. Clap your hands together 20 times and then rub them together until your palms are quite warm.

2. Place your cupped hands over your eyes. Open your eyes and feel the warmth penetrating into them.

3. Rotate the eyes in a circle, first to the right and then to the left. Keep your hands over them.

4. Now uncover your eyes and look up with your eyes, feeling the stretch in your eye muscles. Look down, and to the left and right.

Advanced variation: Make an infinity pattern with your eyes, keeping your head still. After about thirty seconds, reverse direction.

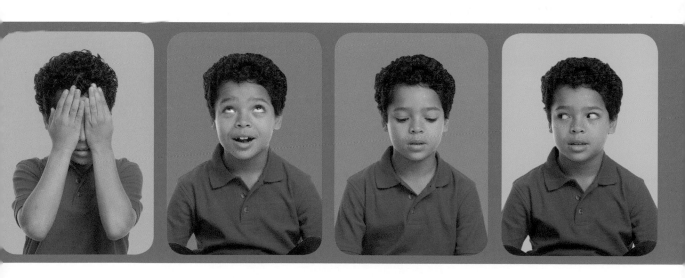

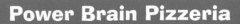

Power Brain Pizzeria

In this exercise, children can learn to relax while experiencing the sense of satisfaction gained from helping others. This can be done with an adult and child pair, as well.

1. Begin by having your partner lie comfortably facedown on the floor. Sit down near your partner. You are the "chef" and your partner is the pizza. Before you begin, pretend to wash your hands by briskly rubbing them together until they are warm.

2. Begin by "kneading the dough," massaging your partner's back and shoulder muscles. Try to use the full hand, without pinching with the fingers.

3. Now pat the dough down with your palms. Cup your hands slightly, patting but not slapping.

4. Sweep your palms on the back to spread the pizza sauce.

5. Then chop the vegetables with the sides of your hands. You can make a fist with your thumbs tucked in or keep your fingers straight.

6. Sprinkle on cheese, tapping your partner with your fingertips.

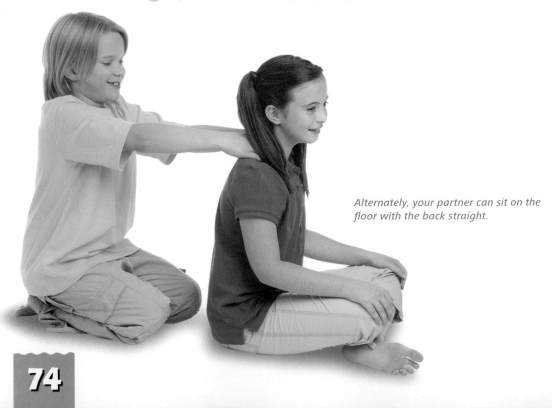

Alternately, your partner can sit on the floor with the back straight.

74

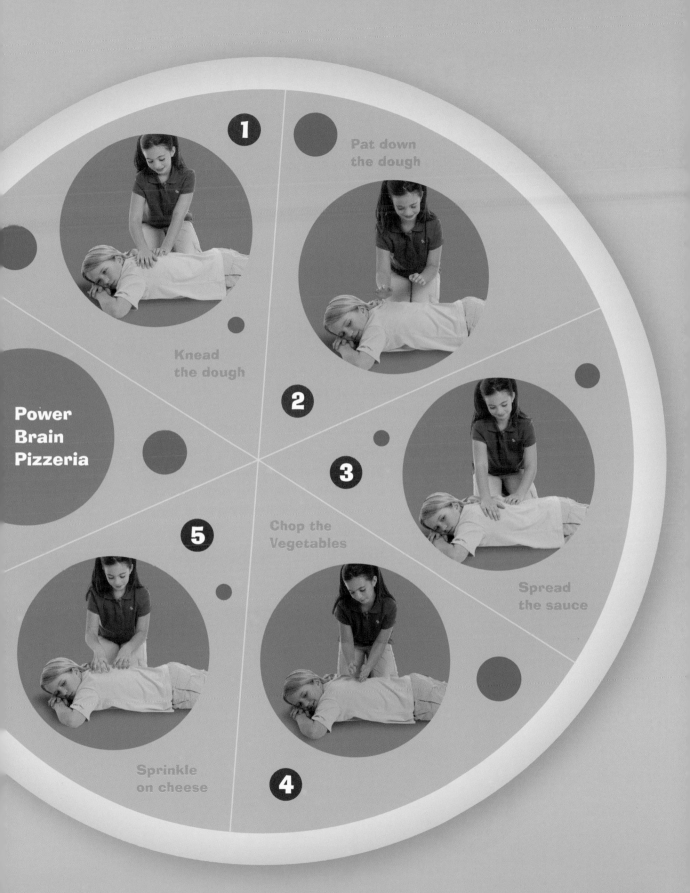

Power
Brain
Pizzeria

1 Knead the dough

Pat down the dough

2

3 Spread the sauce

Chop the Vegetables

5 Sprinkle on cheese

4

Lesson 6
Developing Memory and Focus

Lack of memory is usually something we attribute to older people. When they forget something, we laugh and say they experienced a "senior moment." While it is true that memory skills can decline with age, young people may also lag in that area.

The same environmental conditions that make it difficult to focus also weaken memory skill. Messages and images are constantly flashed before our eyes—in magazines, on billboards, on television, and through the Internet. This constant shower of information makes it very difficult to concentrate and focus solidly. If the brain cannot focus properly on a given task or piece of information, it is unlikely to remember that thing well. Essentially, if the brain cannot easily decide what is worth remembering, much information will be lost.

Furthermore, our memory ability is rarely engaged in today's world. Phone numbers are stored on speed dial, and facts are readily available on the Internet. There is little incentive to remember items that can be easily stored on technological gadgetry. To make up for this deficit, it is important to purposely challenge the memory to keep it sharp.

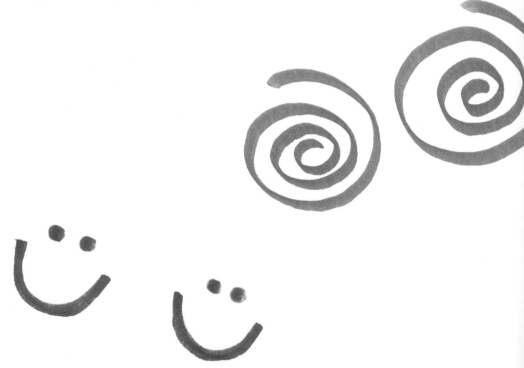

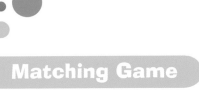

Matching Game

This is a version of the old card-matching game. Even if your child has mastered store-bought versions, they may find the geometric shapes in this version a little more challenging.

Preparation: On one side of thick card stock, draw images of different shapes in various colors—green triangles, orange circles, red squares, etc. Each image will have a matching image on another card to form pairs of matching cards. Draw the images in crayon or some other medium that will not show through on the other side. Alternatively, you can choose pairs of images from computer clip art or photocopied images from magazines to create the cards.

1. Shuffle the cards and place them face down on a table or at various places around the room.

2. Take turns trying to find matching pairs. During a turn, you may flip two cards. If they match, take both cards and try again. If they do not match, the cards must be turned back over and the next person can give it a try. You can see the cards turned over by others and try to remember their locations.

3. The game continues until all matching sets have been revealed. Whoever has the most cards "wins."

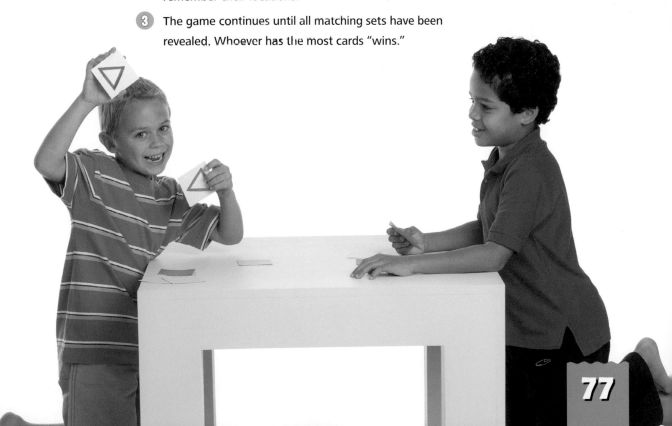

Clapping Games:

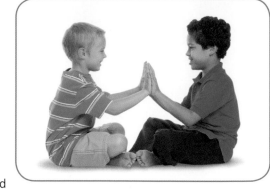

Clapping games such as these are traditionally played by girls in the schoolyard, but they are just as valuable for boys as for girls, as they develop concentration and a sense of rhythm. Try playing these games with your child to pass the time when waiting in line.

1-2-3-2-1 Clapping Game

1 Sit on the floor.

2 Clap your hands once in front of the chest and then once on the floor.

3 Clap once again in front of the chest, and then twice on the floor.

4 Clap once again in front of the chest, and then 3 times on the floor.

5 Now clap once in front of the chest, and twice on the floor.

6 And again, clap once in front of the chest and once on the floor.

7 Continue to follow the 1-2-3-2-1-2-3-2-1 sequence of clapping, seeing how long you can maintain the rhythm. To add a challenge, try slowly increasing the speed.

Alternative: Try this clapping game in pairs, clapping each other's palms instead of the floor.

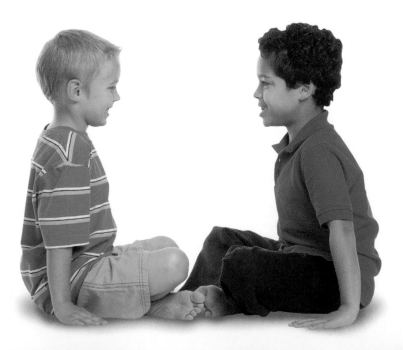

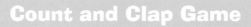

Count and Clap Game

1. Sit or stand across from a partner.

2. Clap once near the chest and then once on your partner's palms.

3. Repeat, but this time clapping twice on your partner's palms.

4. Continue, each time adding another clap on the palms. For maximum concentration, count the numbers silently.

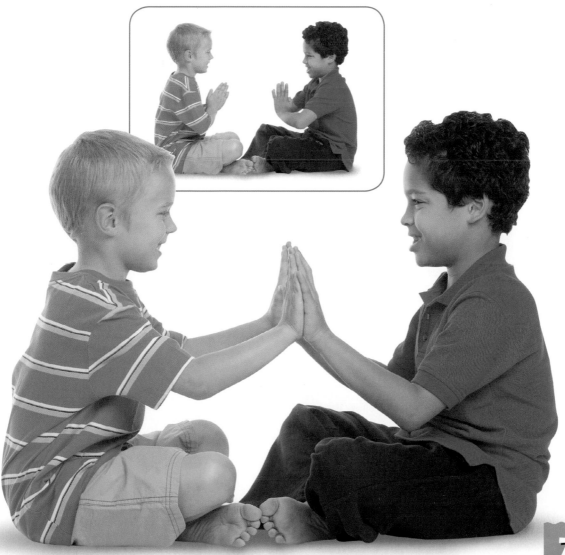

3-6-9 Game

1. Sit or stand across from your partner. Or, if three or more are participating, stand or sit in a circle.

2. Each person counts a number, starting with 1. However, if your number contains a 3, 6, or 9, you must clap instead of saying the number (e.g., 9, 16, 32, etc.). If the number has more than one 3, 6, or 9, or a combination of these numbers (e.g., 66, 93, 36, etc.), you must clap twice.

Energy Ball

Prepare children for this exercise with some stretching (see pages 24–39), chest breathing (see Breathing Buddy exercise, page 71), and deep relaxation (see Lesson 5, pages 71–75) before you begin. This activity is a great way to relax and calm the mind before bed.

1. Sit comfortably with your back straight, preferably in the cross-legged position. Relax your shoulders and tilt your head slightly downward. Place your palms facing upward on the knees.

2. Close your eyes and focus on the surface of the palms. Feel any sensation on the surface of the palms, perhaps tingling or warmth.

3. Gently lift the palms up from the knees and slowly bring the palms closer together until they are about 2 inches apart.

4. Focus on the sensation between the palms. Inhale and slowly draw the hands apart, feeling the sensation growing between the palms. Exhale and feel the "ball" shrink between your hands.

5. Continue to follow the breath as you grow and shrink the energy ball.

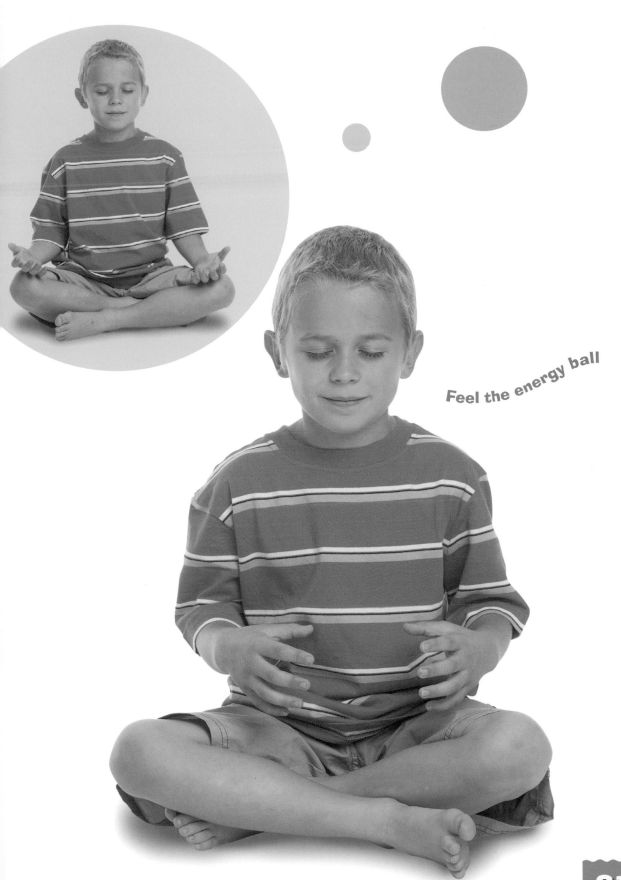

Feel the energy ball

Brain-Body Coordination

Children are in a constant state of flux. Their bodies are always changing, and their minds must struggle to keep up. It is easy for children to feel out of control and uncomfortable in their own skin. As adults, we usually just chalk this up to the "awkward phase" and wait for them to outgrow it.

More physical exercise of all types will help your child gain a sense of centeredness, but strength in the lower body is most important for creating physical stability. Also, moving the arms and legs in opposition across the mid-line of the body helps to establish coordination between the left and right sides of the brain.

Many of the sports and games that children play, such as skateboarding and hopscotch, emphasize balance in movement, and often children become quite proficient at this sort of balancing and coordination. Static balance, the kind of balance needed when you stand still on one foot, requires much more concentrated effort to achieve. Developing this skill calls on the ability to focus deeply while gaining genuine awareness of the entire body as a single entity.

The kind of balancing exercises included in this chapter work not only to balance the body physically but also to balance the mind. As your child learns these postures, new brain connections will naturally be made. Also, improved concentration will come as a natural outgrowth of these exercises.

Balancing Exercises:

Try these exercises to help children develop better balance and focus. Before beginning, have children tap their fingertips gently on their lower abdomen, just below the belly button, to find their center of gravity. Remind them to focus on that point as they attempt to balance.

Tree

1. Stand with your feet together and your palms in the "prayer position."

2. Slowly bring one foot up, placing the bottom of the foot as high as you can on the inner thigh. Push your knee out to the side. (If this is difficult at first, place the foot lower on the leg.)

3. Slowly extend your arms up and out to the side, creating a V shape with your arms.

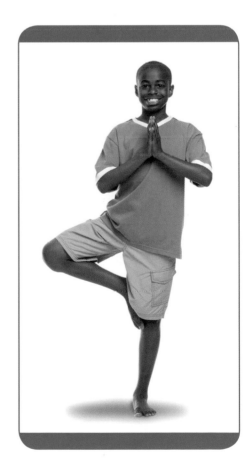

Flamingo

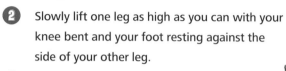

1. Stand with your feet together on the ground and your arms straight out to the side.

2. Slowly lift one leg as high as you can with your knee bent and your foot resting against the side of your other leg.

3. Hold the position for 10 counts. Switch legs and try again.

Later, attempt to hold for up to 30 seconds.

Advanced alternative: Try this with your eyes closed.

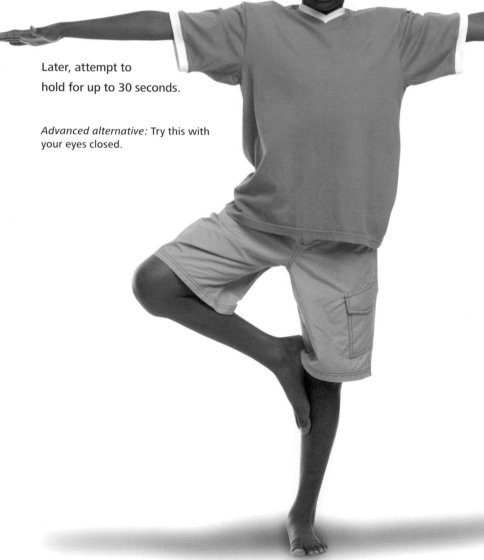

Airplane

1 Bend the body forward, placing the hands on the ground. Knees may be slightly bent.

2 Slowly lift your arms straight out to the side as you lift one of your legs straight back.

3 Slowly straighten the balancing leg. Keep your body bent forward at a 90-degree angle, your arms out to the side, and the other leg straight out. Hold for 10 counts.

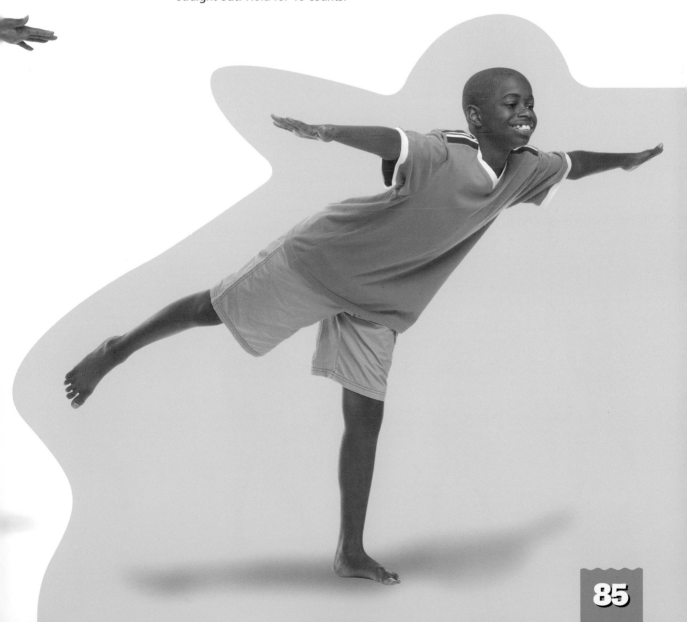

Spiral Dance

This exercise is difficult to follow at first, but it helps to develop coordination of brain hemispheres. It also moves and flexes all the joints and muscles of the body.

1 Hold a small paper plate in your right hand. Hold it on the palm or fingertips without using the fingers to grasp the plate.

2 Slowly bend the arm inward under the armpit. Keeping the palm upward with the plate balanced on it, swing the arm back and up over the head, creating a spiral motion. Move hips as needed to facilitate the movement.

3 Return to the original position, using a downward spiral motion. Repeat 5–10 times.

4 Switch the paper plate to the left hand and begin the same spiraling movement on the left side. Repeat 5–10 times. Switch direction and repeat 5–10 times.

Advanced alternate: When the movement is fairly fluid on both sides, place a paper plate on both hands and try completing the movement simultaneously on both sides.

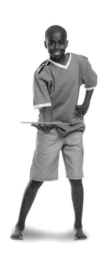
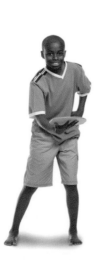
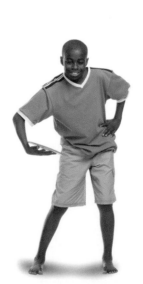
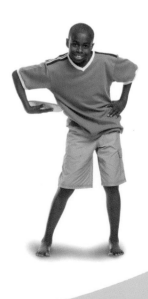

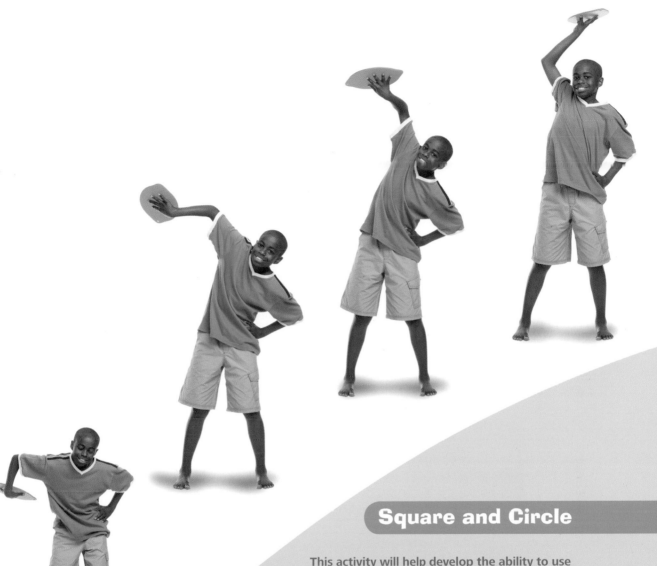

Square and Circle

This activity will help develop the ability to use the right and left hands simultaneously, which requires coordination of the right and left hemispheres of the brain. The activities in Lesson 4 (pages 67–69) are helpful for this as well.

1. Draw a large square on half of a piece of paper and a circle on the other half.

2. With a crayon held in each hand, trace the square with one hand while simultaneously tracing the circle with the other hand.

3. After a few minutes, turn the paper upside down and do it again, using the other hand for each shape.

Balloon Bounce

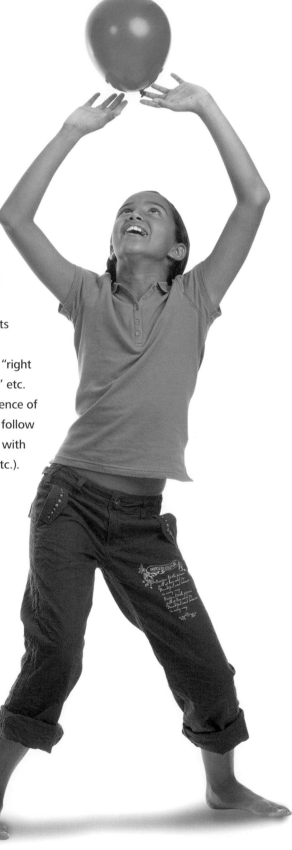

This game really gets kids moving while developing quick thinking and coordination. It works well with one child, but it can also work very well with a large group.

1 Bounce an air-filled balloon from one child to another.

2 Call out names of body parts that the children must use to hit the balloon. Call out, "right elbow," "left knee," "head," etc. Alternatively, create a sequence of movements that they must follow (e.g., bouncing the balloon with the shoulder, hand, knee, etc.). The more body parts you add, the more complicated it becomes.

3 Assign a number to each child. When that number is called, the child must hit the balloon. To make the game more challenging, assign more than one number to each child.

Lesson 8
Emotional Self-Control

As the years pass, children must learn to handle the many emotions that are part of growing up. The process is made all the more difficult if family life is strained or if peer relations are uncomfortable. As much as they would like to, adults cannot wholly prevent the tears, fights, and frustrations that are an inevitable part of life.

However, we can provide a sense of empowerment over the ebb and flow of the mind. Children must know that feelings do not come from outside themselves. We say, "This makes me happy" or "That makes me mad," but in reality, emotions come from within ourselves, from inside our brain. To take full ownership of the brain, it is essential to master the emotions as much as possible. This, of course, can be difficult, since emotions are almost impossible to turn on or off at will. It is vital, however, to gain control of our mind if we wish to pursue a life that is truly creative, peaceful, and productive.

Emotions also have a profound effect on the brain's ability to learn, primarily because the emotional centers of the brain are very closely related to those that govern memory. A negative emotional state can make it difficult, if not impossible, to learn. Negative emotional memories associated with a particular learning experience can influence a person's ability to learn well into adulthood, as the phenomenon of "math anxiety" suggests.

Children are at an advantage, though, when it comes to emotions, because they can change emotional states more quickly and readily than adults. Usually, the younger the child, the more quickly the emotional state can change. For example, think of the toddler who is in a screaming, red-faced tantrum one minute and then is laughing and giggling ten minutes later. Older children hold emotional states longer, but they are similarly resilient—the schoolyard traumas of one day are quite often forgotten the next.

These exercises are designed to help provide balance and stability by calming the emotional swings that are so often disruptive in the child's life. Children can learn how to identify and let go of emotional states, while gaining skills to cope with them. The exercises can also help reveal and alleviate lingering emotional traumas and promote a trusting, loving attitude.

Emotional Inventory

The first step toward emotional control is simply recognizing emotions as they exist. Also, talking about emotions is a good way to start controlling them. In this activity, children are asked to recall emotions they have felt.

1 Ask your child to remember the many emotions that exist—anger, sadness, jealousy, and so on. Look at the pictures provided on this page and ask, "What emotions are these children feeling?"

2 Then ask the child, "What emotions have you felt today?" Have the child show a face or bodily posture that illustrates the emotion. Then go further back in time. "What did you feel yesterday or the day before?" Have older children write down a list of emotions they have felt.

The Smiling Brain

Have you ever heard the old axiom "Smile and the whole world smiles with you"? As it turns out, this is literally true. Sophie Scott, Ph.D., and her team at University College London's Institute of Cognitive Neuroscience have documented that when people hear the sound of laughter, areas of the brain associated with smiling and laughing are activated. Even though they have nothing in particular to smile or laugh about, people are happier when exposed to the expressions of happy people *(see Warren)*.

You don't have to wait for other people to make you happy, either. Just the simple act of smiling itself activates areas in the brain related to feelings of contentedness and joy. Since stress and prolonged negative emotion can have a detrimental effect on the brain, Brain Education recommends making a deliberate effort to smile and laugh, even when it seems like there is nothing worth smiling and laughing about!

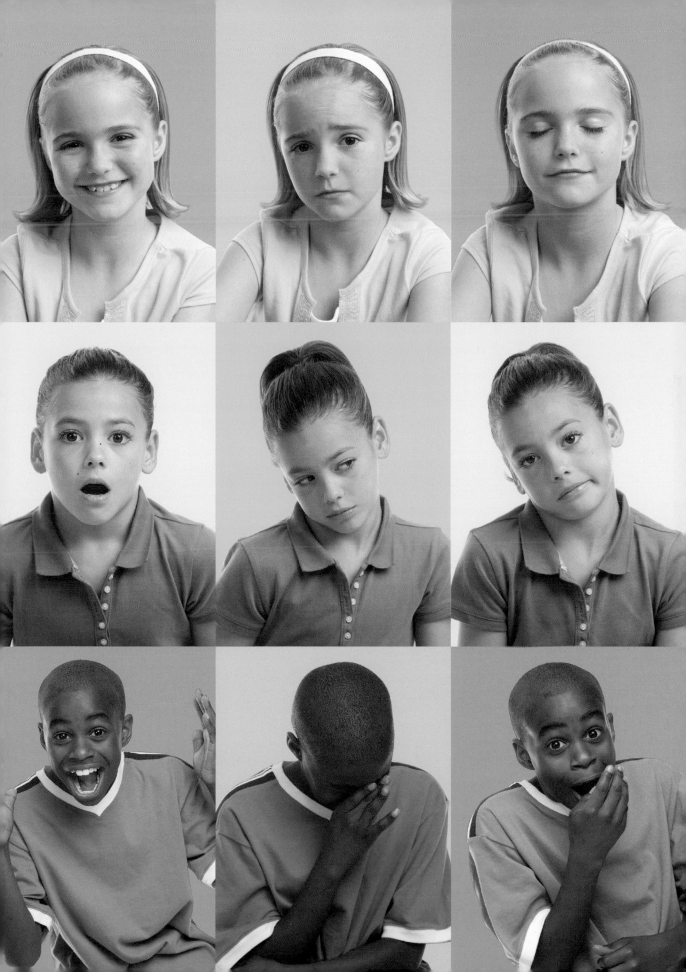

Happy Face/Angry Face

This exercise is designed to introduce the idea that kids can choose what emotions to feel. It will also help them let go of past negative emotions.

1. Remember a time when you felt very angry or unhappy. Tell about that time, and then blow up a balloon, imagining that all the anger is going into the balloon.

2. Tie up your "angry" balloon and draw an unhappy face on it with a permanent felt-tip marker.

3. Now remember a time when you were very happy. Blow the happiness into a second balloon.

4. Tie the "happy" balloon. Using the marker, draw a happy face on the balloon.

5. How does each balloon make you feel when you look at it? Pop the one you least prefer.

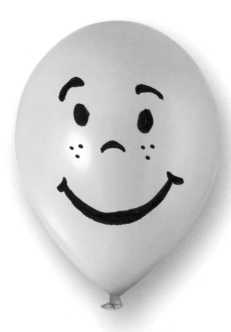
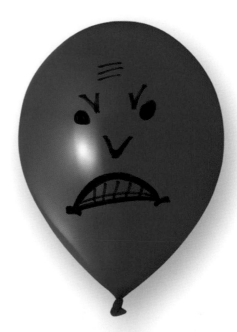

Eye Gaze

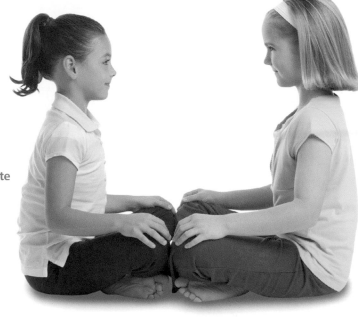

This game is great for parents and other family members to play with children. It helps create openness, overcomes shyness, and promotes self-awareness.

1. Sit down with a partner on the floor. Sit cross-legged with your knees touching. Hold hands.

2. Look directly into each other's eyes for 3 minutes. If this is uncomfortable or culturally inappropriate, just close your eyes and hold hands.

3. Take turns sharing what you felt with each other.

Crazy Laughing Exercise

This exercise is simple—just laugh as hard as you can for one full minute. Research has shown that laughing and smiling have a profoundly positive influence on our health *(see Takahashi)*. Brain chemistry is improved immediately when a person smiles, even when there seems to be no reason to smile!

At first, some children may feel self-conscious about this game. Allow many chances to try. Let the child lie on the floor to flail arms and legs and beat on the ground. And be sure to laugh along with the child!

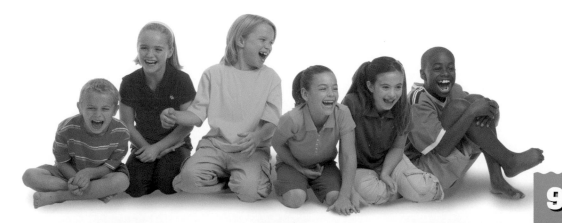

Cultivating Confidence

In many aspects of life, self-confidence is the deciding factor in determining success or failure. Without confidence, we can hardly take a single step in the direction of our dreams, much less actually achieve them. Furthermore, lack of belief in oneself usually translates into lack of belief in other people and the world in general.

Childhood is perhaps the most important time to build confidence. Psychologists often cite childhood trauma as the source of low self-esteem and lack of confidence. So use this important time to help your child understand the importance of personal strength and self-acceptance.

Begin by changing "I can't" attitudes to "I can" attitudes. Children, like adults, may tend to set aside learning new tasks if they do not come easily and automatically to them. This is a really unfortunate choice for the brain, which thrives on learning new things and making new connections. When your children say they don't know how to do something, say to them, "Ask your brain." If it is humanly possible to do something, you can simply ask your brain for the way that is right for it to learn. Guide children to understand that the limitations we put on ourselves are created only in our minds, and we can always find a way to break through those limits.

Finally, remember to teach your children that failure is not a negative thing. It is a normal part of anyone's learning process, and, unless you quit, it is only a temporary state on the path to success. In fact, the ability to cope with and face our own failures may reflect the ultimate kind of confidence.

Flying Eagle

This may be a difficult exercise, but it builds both physical and mental strength.

1. Stand with your feet shoulder width apart, knees slightly bent.

2. Lift your arms up and out to the side, forming 90-degree angles. Turn your palms up so that your palms face the outside.

3. Hold this position for as long as you can, starting with five minutes and working up to 20 minutes.

Identity Drawing

Confidence begins with a solid sense of identity and purpose. Help your child examine that creatively.

Have your child draw a picture of his or her life. Be sure to include all the important details—family, friends, pets, etc. Use more than one piece of paper if you need to, but limit the time to 15 minutes. Ask the child to explain the picture and why certain details were included or left out. Then ask, "What would you change if you could?"

I-Am Declaration

This exercise is especially effective whenever children seem frustrated by some task or situation. It helps them learn to keep looking forward to pushing through obstacles.

1. Ask your child, "Who do you want to be?" The answer could be about their dreams for their adult life, for next week, or even for the next minute.

2. Now shout this dream in one clear, concise, declarative sentence. Make sure the sentence is definite, as in, "I AM strong," not "I want to become strong." Make sure this is yelled as loudly as possible.

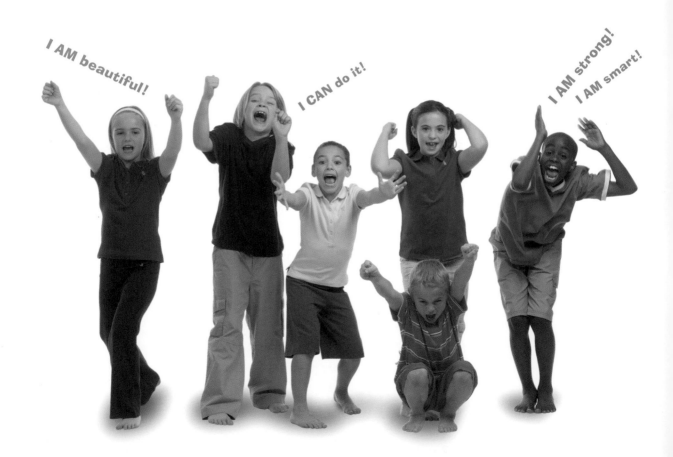

I AM beautiful!

I CAN do it!

I AM strong!

I AM smart!

Unleashing Imagination & Creativity

Adults often complain that kids don't use their imagination as they used to. Their days are packed with preplanned activities—school, sports, tutoring, etc.—and every spare moment is filled in with DVDs, children's cable television programming, and video games. Little time is left to explore the world and create adventures for themselves.

Why should they bother accessing their imagination when our media culture provides computer-animated dinosaurs, battling spaceships, and instantaneous travel to every part of the globe? When these things disappear, the inevitable cry of "I'm bored!" follows.

A bored child is a child who has not learned to draw on the vast creative resources that lie within the brain. A child's mind, once awakened to its own imagination, can produce images and ideas that easily rival those of the Walt Disneys and Steven Spielbergs of this world. In addition, a child's expressions of creativity provide a link to his or her inner workings.

Essentially, a drawing, a skit, or a poem is a reflection of the creator's mental and spiritual state. Through this kind of expression, children release much of the discomfort and pressure of growing up, and they can learn to imagine a world that is better for themselves and everyone around them.

Music Drawing

This exercise encourages kids to "feel" music deeply and to express themselves spontaneously.

1. Gather three stylistically distinct instrumental songs. For example, you might have a lighthearted polka, a soft lullaby, or a booming orchestral piece.

2. Sit comfortably with eyes closed, quietly listening to one of the songs. Notice any colors or feelings that come to mind.

3. Gather crayons whose colors best seem to represent the song.

4. Now play the song again, this time "drawing it." Let your hand move freely in response to the music. Do the same for the other two songs.

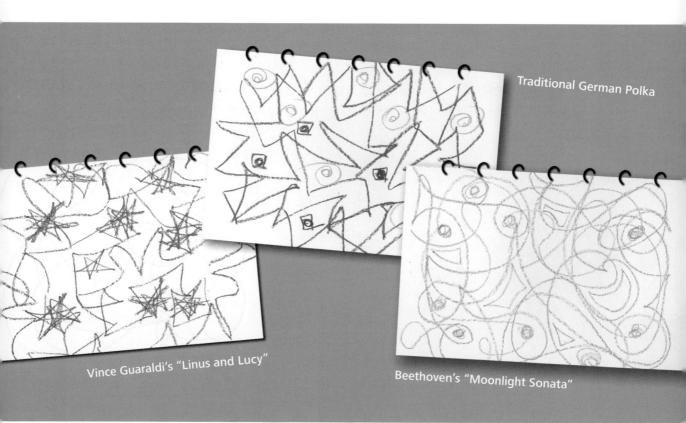

Traditional German Polka

Vince Guaraldi's "Linus and Lucy"

Beethoven's "Moonlight Sonata"

Butterfly Story

Use the story on the following pages to help illustrate creativity and its connection to personal transformation. How you use it may depend on your child's age and pre-ferences. You can choose from one or more of the options below or find some other creative way of using the story.

1. Read the story at bedtime, with soft, lilting music in the background.

2. After reading the story, let your child describe a time when he or she felt like the caterpillar.

3. Read the story to your child, but let him or her read the statements made by the caterpillar.

4. Let your child make up his or her own story based on the pictures.

5. Make a script for the story with your child and act it out together.

6. Let the child draw his or her own pictures for the story.

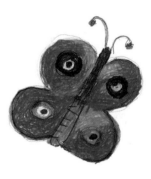

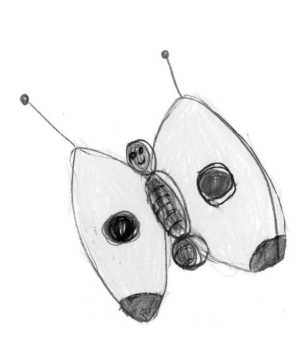

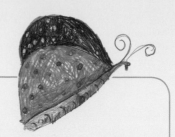

The Butterfly Story...

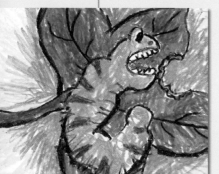

Once upon a time, there lived a group of caterpillars in a great big, green field filled with flowers. Every morning, when the sun came up, they yawned and stretched, and rubbed their fuzzy tummies. **"I'm hungry!"** they would say before taking big, juicy bites of leaves. Then they would slide down the leaves, playing and eating all day.

One day, Baby Caterpillar was taking a sunbath on his leaf when he looked up and saw a beautiful butterfly flying in the sky. "Come fly with me," the butterfly said. "You can fly, too!" But Baby Caterpillar looked at his own short legs and said, **"How can I fly? I don't have any wings!"**

A few days later, Baby Caterpillar's older sister showed him a picture of their father when he was little. She told him a story: "Once, our dad was a baby cater-pillar just like you. One day at caterpillar school, Daddy said, "I'm going to turn into a flying butterfly someday!" All of Daddy's friends pointed at him. "How can you fly?" they asked, laughing. "You don't have any wings! Don't be silly! You can't fly!" But our dad didn't let that bother him. He believed in himself. And what is our father today?" Big Sister asked. **"A butterfly with huge yellow wings!"** sighed Baby Caterpillar. "That's right," said Big Sister, "Dad never gave up on his dream of becoming a butterfly. And now he flies all over the meadow with his beautiful yellow wings!"

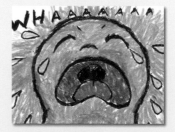

Baby Caterpillar thought, **"My dad believed he could fly. If he did it, then so can I!"** Baby Caterpillar made some wings with leaves, strapped them to his arms, and tried to fly. **"Ahhh!"** he screamed as he fell from the tree.

"Whaaaah!" he cried. **"I want to fly like a butterfly, but I don't**

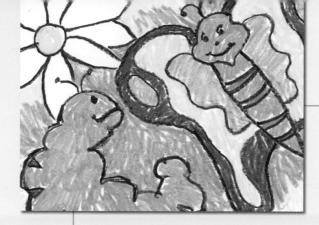

have any wings! Whahah! I wish I could fly!"

One day, Baby Caterpillar's favorite uncle came to visit. **"Uncle,"** he said, **"where did you get those big, beautiful wings?"** Uncle smiled and said, "You also have big, beautiful wings inside of you. You can't see them now, but they are there!" Baby Caterpillar was so happy. **"Will I be able to fly with them?"** he asked. "Yes, you will," said Uncle. "I will teach you!

"Hang on tightly to this vine," said Uncle. "Here we go!" Baby Caterpillar flapped his arms wildly. **"Ugh, ugh…it's too hard…but I really want to fly …I can do it!"** He flapped his arms until they hurt, but he never gave up.

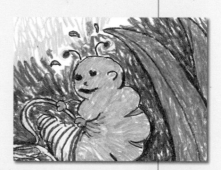

One day, as the weather turned cooler, Baby Caterpillar found that he could pull a string out of his body. He worked very hard, winding the string around his body from the tip of his toes to the top of his head. **"I have to find the wings inside of me. I can do it. I can do it!"** Baby Caterpillar slept in the cocoon, dreaming of the wings he hoped to have.

Three weeks later, Baby Caterpillar slowly opened his cocoon and came out. He looked down at himself and gasped. He wasn't a baby anymore. He had become a beautiful golden butterfly! He knew from then on that he could become any-thing he wanted to be. All he had to do was believe. He smiled, spread his big golden wings, and flew gracefully away.

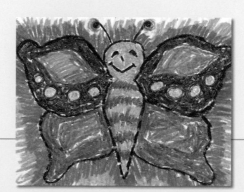

Butterfly Dance

This exercise encourages kids to express themselves through movement. It can also serve as a positive symbolic starting place for any change that may be taking place in their lives. Play some light music that your child can dance to during this exercise.

1. Pretend that you are a little caterpillar, crawling around the room. You love to eat the leaves and watch the grown-up butterflies flying about. What kind of butterfly do you want to be?

2. Now crouch down on the floor in some safe hiding place in the room. Wrap yourself up in a blanket or sheet. This is your cocoon. What does it feel like in the cocoon? Do you want to come out?

3. As the music plays, slowly wriggle out of your cocoon. You are now a little butterfly. How do you feel to be out of your cocoon? Slowly unfold your brand-new wings.

4. Open up your wings and "fly" around the room, feeling and moving to the music. Express what kind of butterfly you are in the way you move.

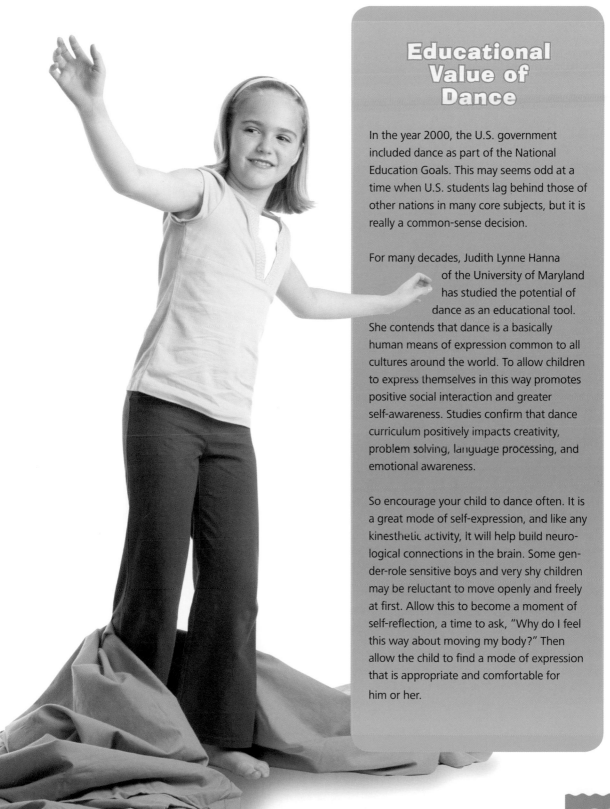

Educational Value of Dance

In the year 2000, the U.S. government included dance as part of the National Education Goals. This may seems odd at a time when U.S. students lag behind those of other nations in many core subjects, but it is really a common-sense decision.

For many decades, Judith Lynne Hanna of the University of Maryland has studied the potential of dance as an educational tool. She contends that dance is a basically human means of expression common to all cultures around the world. To allow children to express themselves in this way promotes positive social interaction and greater self-awareness. Studies confirm that dance curriculum positively impacts creativity, problem solving, language processing, and emotional awareness.

So encourage your child to dance often. It is a great mode of self-expression, and like any kinesthetic activity, it will help build neuro-logical connections in the brain. Some gender-role sensitive boys and very shy children may be reluctant to move openly and freely at first. Allow this to become a moment of self-reflection, a time to ask, "Why do I feel this way about moving my body?" Then allow the child to find a mode of expression that is appropriate and comfortable for him or her.

Lesson 11
Goal Setting for Growth

One of the most common questions adults ask kids is, "What do you want to be when you grow up?" The answer is often something like "a fireman" or "a doctor." Kids seem to instinctively know that we are asking about future career choice, reflecting our notion that the quality of "being" is inextricably linked to how you earn a living.

Perhaps the question "What do you want to be when you grow up?" should also be asked in a deeper and more meaningful sense. Maybe we should also ask, "What sort of character would you like to have? How do you want to feel about yourself? How do you want to treat other people?" These may seem like overly deep, almost burdensome questions to ask a child, but in fact children are making these decisions, whether we ask them directly or not. The child's character and emotional habits are being formed in every encounter and experience. It is on the playground that we decide to live by the fists or by conscience. It is through play that we learn how to keep friends and make enemies.

These aspects of "being" almost certainly have more direct impact on our children's eventual happiness than the amount of money they make or the kind of job they pursue. The definition of "success" based solely on money and career is obviously shallow and incomplete. When a child can envision the kind of person he or she wants to be, and can take action to achieve that goal, he or she will have achieved true brain mastery, the last and most important step in the Brain Education system.

The visualization and goal-setting activities in this lesson can help children become the people they want to be. They have already learned valuable skills of emotional control and creativity. Now they can apply those concepts to begin creating a life picture for themselves. Career and education may be an important part of this picture, but more important is the personal strength of character needed to achieve these goals.

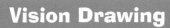

Vision Drawing

Have your child draw a picture of him or herself having achieved some goal he or she would like to attain. It could be becoming a fireman, scoring a goal in soccer, or traveling to another country—anything is fine. Let the child share about the drawing and tell how he or she would like to achieve that goal.

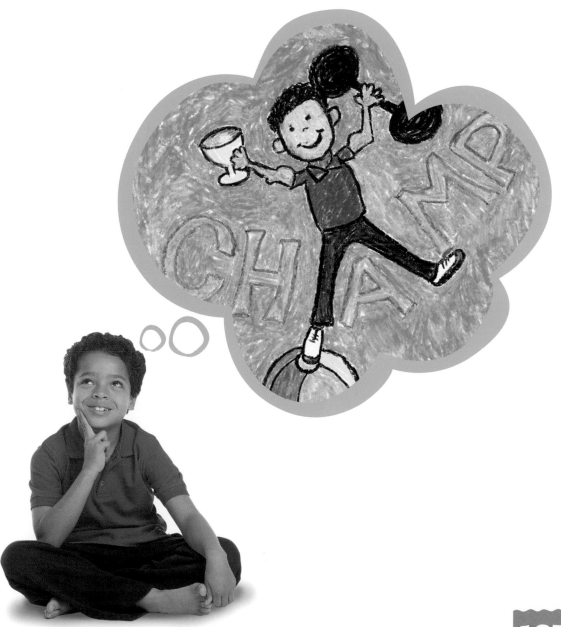

Vision Tree

On a large piece of paper, draw the trunk and branches of a tree. Label the trunk "my life," and label the branches with aspects of life that are important to the child—school, relationships, character, sports, etc. You may leave some branches to fill in later. Then cut out leaves from green construction paper. Write on the leaves any goal the child has—to read a certain book, to change a habit, or to gain a certain skill. Tape or glue the leaves on when the goal has been achieved. Hang the tree on the child's wall and watch it and your child blossom!

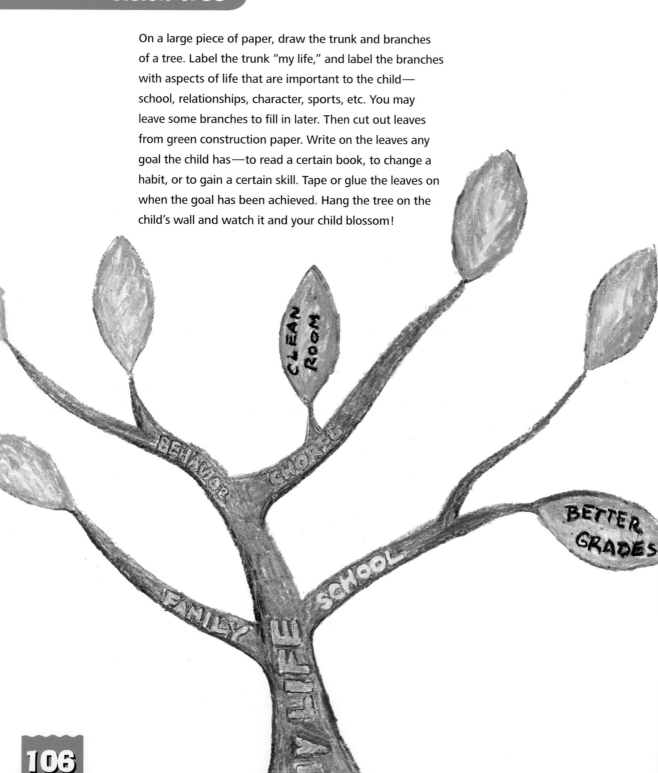

Power Brain Earth Kids

One of the most important decisions for your child will be how to use his or her brain in relation to other brains. Technology has caused the world to effectively "shrink." As a result, children will have to deal with a large variety of cultures and people in their lifetimes. The artificial barriers of political boundaries are breaking down in light of the communication age. In fact, the younger generation may be the first in the history of humanity to identify themselves as citizens of Earth, rather than of a single nation.

Furthermore, environmental concerns are bound to reach their zenith early in the twenty-first century. Our children will likely be required to make very challenging decisions regarding our use of the planet's resources. The human brain becomes all the more important when you consider its effect on the planet.

It is not for us adults to decide how the Earth will be used in the future. But we can help our children connect to and experience the natural world. Young people's lives are often woefully lacking in contact with nature. Out of fear, we rarely let them roam freely, and contacts with the wild world are few and far between. You might ask yourself, "Does my child know the difference between an oak tree and a pine tree? Between a sparrow and a robin?"

Author Richard Louv, in the book *Last Child in the Woods*, contends that many of the behavioral and learning issues that plague kids today are actually the result of something he calls "nature-deficit disorder." Many play experiences these days are "virtual" rather than "real." Essentially, this leads to a kind of spiritual and mental disconnection that creates many problems. For this reason, many psychologists have turned to "nature-play" as a treatment for attention deficit disorders.

So do what you can to reconnect yourself and your children to the joys of nature. There may ultimately be no better medicine for the brain.

Aliens in the Woods

Go to some natural setting, such as a park or wooded area. Ask your child to pretend to be a space alien who has just landed on planet Earth. The alien really wants to experience Earth, but he or she does not have eyes like humans. So you must carefully guide your little alien to experience the wonders of nature. Blindfold the child or have him or her close eyes tight. You can guide the hand to feel the bark of a tree, or pick up a leaf and rub it gently against the cheek. (Watch out for itchy and prickly things!) Instruct the alien to smell a fragrant flower or rub rocks together to make a sound. After a while, switch roles, making the child the human and the adult the alien.

Heal-the-World Meditation

Begin with the Energy Ball activity presented on page 80. Imagine the earth in front of you. What does the Earth look like to you? What do you feel? Now, place the energy ball into the earth. Imagine the Earth glowing. Share with each other what you saw in your mind's eye.

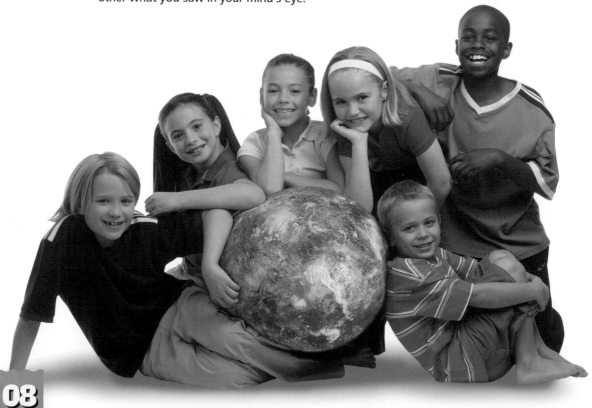

The Journey Continues

The last step of Brain Education is called "Brain Mastery," but that is hardly something that can be accomplished in one series of lessons. Rather, brain mastery is something that must be pursued throughout a lifetime. Your child will continue to face the obstacles and difficulties of life. Sometimes he or she will achieve success, and at other times he or she will experience profound failure. What really matters is how your child faces these things. With the right orientation toward life, he or she can face hardship with undying confidence that the answers to life's problems already exist within his or her brain.

These lessons are not a magic potion that can take away all of your child's troubles and difficulties. But, hopefully, the contents of this book have in some way been magical, in the sense that they have transformed and reoriented your views of your child's abilities and characteristics. Your child is a gift, not only for your life, but also for this world and humanity as a whole. Please continue to look at him or her as a storehouse of limitless potential, for children are the creators of the future, which stretches out before them like an endless canvas. And as a parent who proactively helps your child uncover his or her best qualities and potentials, you are also a timeless, precious gift to all generations yet to come.

Suggestions for Classroom Use

Although this book was written primarily with parents and their children in mind, teachers also will find a great deal of useful material in it. Most of the exercises in this book can be easily adapted for classroom use. You may want to use one lesson every week, or perhaps one per month if that is not possible. The important thing is to make brain awareness part of your classroom culture. If time or curriculum restraints do not allow for integration of full lessons, try using simple exercises to help children focus, or find ways to integrate the exercises into existing lesson plans. Here are some ideas for you:

▶ ## Use BE to build basic skills:

Focus: Itsy Bitsy Brainy (67), Tap and Sweep (67), Circuit Drawing (68), Golden Brain Meditation (72), Matching Game (77), 1-2-3-2-1 Clapping Game (78), Count and Clap (79), 3-6-9 Game (80), Energy Ball (80), Balancing Exercises (82), Square and Circle (87).

Anxiety/stress relief: Body and Brain Relaxation (55), Little Brain Relaxation (65), Circuit Drawing (68), Brain Breathing and Relaxation (70), Emotional Inventory (90), Crazy Laughing Exercise (93), Music Drawing (98).

Memory: Matching Game (77), Count and Clap Game (79), Emotional Inventory (90).

Cooperation: Partner Exercises (38), Power Brain Pizzeria (74), Count and Clap Game (79), Eye Gaze (93), Aliens in the Woods (108).

▶ ## Integrate BE exercises into traditional subject matter:

Language Arts: Brain Watching and Drawing (56), Emotional Inventory (90), Happy Face/Angry Face (92), Eye Gaze (93), Identity Drawing (95), I-Am Declaration (96), Butterfly Story (99), Vision Drawing (105), Vision Tree (106), Heal-the-World Meditation (108), Aliens in the Woods (108).

Mathematics: 1-2-3-2-1 Clapping Game (78), Count and Clap Game (79), 3-6-9 Game (80).

Science: Play-doh Brains (54), Brain Watching and Drawing (56), Little Brain Game (58), Little Brain Relaxation (65), Aliens in the Woods (108).

Art/ Music Appreciation: Play-doh Brains (54), Brain Watching and Drawing

(56), Circuit Drawing (68), Square and Circle (87), Happy Face/Angry Face (92), Identity Drawing (95), Music Drawing (98), Butterfly Story (99), Butterfly Dance (102), Vision Drawing (105), Vision Tree (106).

Physical Education: Brain-Body Activation (24–39), Body and Brain Check-up (43), BE Push-ups (49), BE Sit-ups (50), Sleeping Tiger Power Builder (51), Little Brain Exercises (60), Bright Eyes Exercise (73), Balancing Exercises (82), Spiral Dance (86), Balloon Bounce (88), Flying Eagle (95), Butterfly Dance (102).

▶ ## Use BE games as an incentive for students to finish difficult tasks:

Fun Stuff: Partner Exercises (38), Play-doh Brains (54), Breathing Buddy Exercise (71), Power Brain Pizzeria (74), Matching Game (77), Clapping Games (78), Balloon Bounce (88), Crazy Laughing Exercise (93), Music Drawing (98), Butterfly Dance (102), Aliens in the Woods (108).

Benefits in the classroom:

- Relieves test anxiety
- Builds good interpersonal relationships
- Boosts energy level or refocuses the class
- Creates cooperative classroom environment
- Improves student-teacher relationship
- Encourages physical health
- Stimulates creativity

Contributed by BE and elementary school instructor David Beal.

Brain Education for Enhanced Learning

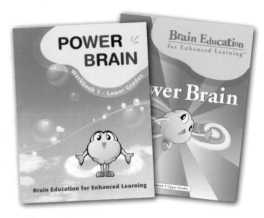

Brain Education is also available in a comprehensive program for schools, called Brain Education for Enhanced Learning. This deeply experiential program is designed to work with schools' existing curricula to promote productive functioning of the body and brain.

Through the Brain Education for Enhanced Learning program, students may:

- Enhance physical well-being and self-efficacy
- Learn basic skills for stress management
- Increase attention span
- Develop social skills, such as trust and cooperation
- Harness the power of imagination and creativity

The program is modular and fully customizable to suit the needs of any school's educational objectives. Implementation of the program includes intensive teacher training and continuous support of qualified BE staff members. The program activities are supported by grade-appropriate workbooks and a detailed teacher's manual. If you are considering Brain Education for Enhanced Learning for your school, please contact:

PowerBrain Education, LLC
340 Jordan Road
Sedona, AZ 86336
T) 928-203-0840
info@powerbrainedu.com
www.powerbrainedu.com

Endorsements

▶ **From Educators**

"Interweaving Brain Education activities throughout the curriculum provides alternative ways to improve the academic performance of students and educate them to care for their emotional well-being."

—**Susana Nakamoto-Gonzalez, Ph.D.**
Professor, Golden West College | Huntington Beach, CA

"I had Brain Education adopted as a regular class for children who often got caught fighting and who were easily distracted. I saw remarkable transformations in children who previously seemed to give up on everything. These children now had restored energy and confidence in their eyes."

—**Diana Anton**
Cluster Coordinator, Near North Magnet | Chicago, IL

"[My Brain Education trained kindergarteners] seemed to transform from wild and crazy in September to energetic and focused by the end of May. By the end of the year they were much more comfortable with their bodies and abilities."

—**Gail M. Olson**
Administrator, Sedona Montessori School | Sedona, AZ

"This book is wonderful and revolutionary. *Power Brain Kids* is congruent with the holistic view of education—to help facilitate, support and expand the growth of all persons in their experience of life."

—**Rosemary White Shield, Ph.D.**
Professor, Iowa State University | Ames, IA

▶ **From Children**

"I figured out a lot of things I didn't know about myself. I think Brain Education made me believe more in myself…that I can do something if I set my mind to it and if I can keep telling myself that I can do it."

—**Lisa Ekenbanger, age 12**

"The things that improved after doing Brain Education are my studies and my ability to concentrate. I am less distracted."

—**Michael Stevens, age 11**

Index

References

Dennison, Dr. Paul E. *Edu-K for Kids.* Ventura: Edu-Kinesthetics, 1987.

————. *Brain Gym.* Ventura: Edu-Kinesthetics, 1986.

Gottman, John. *Raising Emotionally Intelligent Children.* New York: Simon and Schuster, 1998.

Hannaford, Carla. *The Dominance Factor: Knowing Your Dominant Eye, Ear, Brain, Hand, and Foot.* Alexander: Great Ocean, 1997.

————. *Smart Moves: Why Learning Is All in Your Head.* Salt Lake City: Great River Books, 1995.

Hanna, Judith Lynne. *Partnering Dance and Education: Intelligent Moves for Changing Times.* Champaign: Human Kinetics, 1999.

Louv, Richard. *The Last Child in the Woods: Saving Our Children from Nature-Deficit Disorder.* Chapel Hill: Algonquin, 2006.

Nunley, Kathie F. *Layered Curriculum: The Practical Solution for the Teachers with More than One Student in Their Classroom.* 2nd ed. Brains.org, 2004.

Promislow, Sharon. *Making the Brain Body Connection.* Vancouver: Enhanced Learning and Integration, 2005.

Takahashi, Kiyotake, et al. *"Effects of Laughter on Immune Function."* *International Journal of Molecular Medicine.* December, 2001.

Vail, Priscilla L. *Emotion: The On/Off Switch for Learning.* Cambridge: Modern Learning Press, 1993.

Warren, J., et al. *"Positive Emotions Preferentially Engage Auditory-Motor 'Mirror' System."* *Journal of Neuroscience.* December 12, 2006.

Acknowledgments

Special thanks to the following people for all they have done and continue to contribute:

BE Instructors
Nora Lee
Warrington Parker
Brenda Parker
Tia Robinson
Penny Perel Costanzo
Anne Cowardin-Bach
Nancy Bigelow
David Beal
Sheran Mattson
Geoffrey Leigh

Editors
Nicole Dean
Bernard W. Silver
Karen Stough

Photographer
Paul Markow

Designers
Melanie Pantell
Joseph Cortese

Production Manager
Ji-In Kim

Models
Brickel Peters
Devan Ingram
Henry Reed
Ian Reed
John Duffy
Kealey Bride
Kendall Glover
Shelby Irwin

About the Author

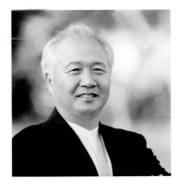

For the past twenty-five years, author Ilchi Lee has dedicated his life to finding ways to develop the potential of the human brain. Brain Education, a mind-body training program that helps unlock the brain's true potential, is the primary fruit of his search. Through numerous programs for adults and children, many thousands of people have discovered a path to greater health, happiness, and peace.

The ultimate purpose of brain development, according to Lee, is lasting world peace. His "Brain-Peace Philosophy" identifies the brain as the seat of human consciousness, and therefore it is through developing the brain that humanity can transcend its destructive patterns.

Lee's quest to bring healing to humanity began in the 1980s when he started teaching a single student in a Korean park. The student, a stroke victim, improved dramatically, and many more people gathered to discover the training system Lee had developed from ancient traditional methods. Eventually, the first Dahn Center opened, which blossomed into a network of over six hundred centers worldwide.

Currently, Lee serves as the president of the International Graduate University for Peace. Also, he is president of the Korean Institute of Brain Science and chairman of the International Brain Education Association. Lee is the author of twenty-nine books. His work as a peacemaker and educator has been widely recognized, both in his native Korea and in the international community.

Also by This Author

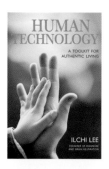

Human Technology

Ilchi Lee presents a toolkit for self-reliant management of the core issues of life: health, family, and life purpose. Meditation, breath-work, and Oriental healing arts are offered as personal health management skills. A distinctive perspective on relationships and an inspirational guide to discover one's passionate life purpose are featured. This book also includes a practical guide to optimize our life's master controller—the brain.

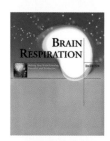

Brain Respiration

The human brain is the nexus for the meeting of body, mind, and spirit. Through conscious practice of Brain Respiration, you will develop a "power brain" that may be characterized as creative, peaceful, and productive. This b ook provides you with the principles and methodology of Brain Respiration.

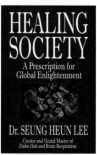

Healing Society

Ilchi Lee's first book released in English reached #1 in amazon.com overall sales ranking within a month of publication. The author emphasizes throughout the book that enlightenment is not just for a select few, but available to everyone. This book includes stories of the author's personal experiences in his quest to find the meaning of life.

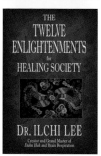

The Twelve Enlightenments for Healing Society

Ilchi Lee offers readers the practical tools to "stop seeking enlightenment and start acting it." He shows readers how to become what he calls "enlightened activists" and push past the artificial boundaries that prevent us from realizing we are all members of a single human society.